Gluten Free Cookbook

Gluten Free Weight Loss for Gluten Free Living

Laura Roberts and Janet Gonzales

Table of Contents

APPETIZERS, SIDE DISHES AND SOUPS 153

BREAKFAST 175

Introduction

This book is perfect for anyone that has to live with gluten allergies or intolerances. The symptoms of gluten intolerances alone are terrible. The discomfort brought on just from consuming gluten is enough to make you want to change your diet completely. Some need to eat gluten free out of necessity. Some will eat gluten free because they wish to change their dieting to one that promises to be healthier. People with the gluten issues will find relief when they simply exclude any foods with gluten from their diet. This book offers all the recipes as gluten free and gives you enough choices to plan menus for weeks in advance if you pull recipes from both sections.

In order to make any dieting successful you need to prepare your body first. Unless you are already on the gluten free diet and you purchased this book for the recipe choices you should read on. Below will be advice on how to make dieting a success for you.

Make sure you get plenty of rest. You may wonder what this has to do with dieting and it has plenty to do with it. A body that is not well rested will think it is in stress and the digestive system reacts. The body tends to hold onto calories and fat longer if it is in stress. You can remedy this by simply trying to get a good night's rest every night. You need about six to eight hours of sleep a night. Some people may need more while others may need less. It depends. You know what your sleep level is. So make sure when you wake up in the morning you are not groggy for half of the day. If you are then add more sleep at night. Try to take naps - a 20 minute nap will recharge you. Take breaks throughout the day, just 10 minutes here and there to rest your eyes and it will work wonders. And it will work wonders on your body and your digestive system.

Something that should already be a good habit is drinking plenty of water a day. While you can get your "water" from drinking tea and fruit juice, you still should drink enough plain water too. Eight cups of water a day is quite a bit, if you drank two cups with each meal you would have to drink an additional two more between meals. Keep this in mind so you make sure to get all the water you need. You can figure out exactly how much water you need by taking your weight in pounds and dividing in half and this is the amount of water you need to drink per day. For example, if you weigh 130 pounds, divide that by 2 and you have 65. You would drink 65 ounces of water per day.

If you have bad habits like smoking, drinking, taking recreational drugs or even to junk foods, you should try to break these bad habits to make a complete change in lifestyle to a healthy one. Breaking bad habits can take up to three weeks or longer. If you need assistance with breaking them, seek advice from your health care provider. Wean from the junk food by replacing the junk food with a nutritious snack every several days, and do this for three weeks solid. By the time you get to the third week your body should be craving the healthy foods and not the junk food. The same goes for caffeine. Just cut back a drink every week until you are at zero. Speak with your health care provider about the caffeine; it may be okay to have one or two drinks a day.

The next habit you need to make is to exercise, unless you already do it. Exercise is very beneficial for everybody. It is especially beneficial to aid in weight loss as well. Adding exercise to your lifestyle is vital to helping your body to be at its healthiest. If you have been diagnosed with high cholesterol, hypertension, and or high blood glucose levels, then diet combined with exercise is one of the best treatments. Most doctors agree that when these three are diagnosed the first line of treatment is to eat right and exercise.

Exercise routines do not need to be too strenuous in order to do the body good. In fact, doing slow and steady exercises will do the body as good as if you spend a half an hour doing high impact aerobics. You can spend 10 minutes stretching, 10 minutes at a light walk / jog, and then finish with 10 more minutes of stretching to do your body good. In truth it only takes a half an hour of honest exercise, where you are moving the entire time (or stretching) to be sufficient. And this needs to be done only every other day. You may get to where you enjoy exercising and may wish to increase the time or intensity. This is okay too as long as you keep it in moderation.

The key to dieting success is balance and moderation. If you have a specific need like a gluten intolerance then you must adhere to the strict guidelines and avoid gluten. If you do not and you just want to change the way you eat or want to lose weight, you can adapt to this diet slowly. You can choose from both sides of the book and enjoy home cooked meals that are gluten free.

Feel free to combine the recipes and create your own dishes. You have enough recipes in this book to plan your menu for several weeks without repeating a meal. Add in food like fresh fruit and vegetables to give you all the fiber you need. If you have any questions or concerns about the gluten free diet seek the advice of your health care provider, especially if you suffer from any health ailments or are on prescription medications.

Section 1: Gluten Free Diet

If you have read any magazine or newspaper, seen any television commercial or used the internet lately, you have likely heard or read something about a gluten free diet. But just what is gluten free? Simply put, gluten free diet is a diet that excludes gluten, the primary villain for those who have celiac disease. However, many people have found that eliminating gluten from their diet also helps with allergies, certain autism characteristics (although there is some controversy over these claims) and even weight loss.

Gluten is a protein that is found in many grains including wheat, rye and barley. It can cause all sorts of problems with people who have gluten sensitivity or celiac disease. For people with celiac disease, it can cause quite a bit of discomfort, creating inflammation in the small intestines. Other symptoms of celiac disease include irritability, fatigue, decreased appetite, chronic (sometimes bloody) diarrhea and growth problems (in children). For individuals living with this condition, a gluten free diet can be a godsend.

There is some concern among doctors that a gluten free diet can be linked to certain nutrient deficiencies. Many prepared products and are gluten free are not enriched or fortified with nutrients like fiber, folate and iron. Most traditional breads and cereals are enriched and fortified with these nutrients so some people may not realize the disconnect. Additionally, gluten free foods may not always be available, leaving patients to omit vital foods from their diets, thus failing to consume the number of grain servings that are recommended daily.

The menus and meal plans in this book are well rounded and nutritionally sound. Every effort was make to ensure that the recipes here have ingredients that should be fairly easy to find. And when you must alter your diet, the easier it is to find the ingredients and foods you need, the easier it is to stick with the plan. Being gluten free is important for those who require that special diet, but getting the proper nutrition is equally important.

Gluten Free Diet Basics

Beginning a gluten free diet requires some forethought and planning. We are bombarded with gluten rich foods every day in many of our most common foods (like bread and pasta) so cutting it out can require you to make some adjustments to your diet and lifestyle. At first glance it may look like you have to cut out a lot of foods. In reality, you just have to shift things around a bit – most of the time anyway. You will have to change the way you do some things like shop and cook.

You will have to learn how to read and understand labels. The most current research regarding celiac disease suggests that the safe level of gluten in a finished product is about 200 parts per million (ppm), or 0.02% or less. However, it could even go as low as 20 parts per million, or 0.002%. These are the maximum levels of gluten that are considered safe for people with celiac disease.

While food labels vary from country to country, in the United States, the Food and Drug Administration (FDA) has no set guidelines governing the labeling of gluten free foods. Currently, manufacturers are not required to disclose gluten containing ingredients on their labeling.

Additionally, foods labeled "gluten free" may not be entirely gluten free. The FDA currently allows "trace" amounts of gluten in foods that are labeled gluten free. There are proposals on the table to improve the labeling of gluten free foods, but at the publication of this book, no finalizations to this proposal have been made and no final decision is in sight. "Trace" amounts, per the FDM means that it allows a variance of a supposedly small, but undefined amount. However, the majority of manufacturers are adhering to the proposed regulations indicating that gluten free labeled products contain less than 20 ppm.

Another significant concern when purchasing foods labeled gluten free is cross contamination. Again, labeling for cross contamination is very poor. When shopping for gluten free products, you must be careful because some grains, flours and seeds that are inherently gluten free but not labeled as such are actually contaminated with gluten. This could cause you to accidentally ingest gluten even though you are trying to maintain a gluten free diet.

Cross contamination can occur at any stage of the processing and preparation of a food. For instance, a gluten free food that is going through the manufacturing process may become contaminated with gluten if that machinery is also used to processed foods containing gluten. But even your own home is not exempt. If you use a toaster for bread containing gluten, then you can easily contaminate your gluten free bread if you put it in that same toaster. It is very important to keep gluten free foods and foods containing gluten separate including storage, preparation and cooking.

When you are shopping, read the ingredients list even if the food is normally considered a gluten free food. Gluten can be found in a variety of ingredients such as modified food starch, vegetable proteins, barley of wheat derivatives, malt flavoring and starch. Ingredients like dextrin, maltodextrine may also contain gluten unless they are labeled as corn malt. Dextrose, however, is considered to be a gluten free food regardless of its source because it is so highly modified.

Gluten Free Food Basics

The healthiest diet is all natural with no processed foods. This is actually very compatible with a gluten free diet.

Beans, nuts and seeds

Beans, nuts and seeds are gluten free if you consume them in their natural state. Once they are processed or have a bunch of fancy seasonings added in they may lose their gluten free status. Always read the labels!

Lean protein

Fresh, lean beef, fresh eggs, poultry, shrimp and fish are great choices. Just make sure that you don't opt for batter coated, marinated or breaded versions of these foods. Just watch out for cross contamination. Check out the food prep area if you can or ask someone behind the counter if any of the products are cut, packaged or prepared in the same area or using the same equipment as breads or other gluten products.

Sausage can be very tricky. Many manufacturers use

bread crumbs as a filler so make sure that the package specifies gluten free. Chicken sausage and beef sausage can be very nice compliments to your menu. You can also typically find gluten free deli meats fairly easily, but check out the prep area at the deli counter to avoid cross contamination from shared slicing equipment.

Fruits and vegetables

Fruits and vegetables are naturally gluten free – when consumed in their natural form. Processed foods may become cross contaminated or may contain additives that have gluten so read your labels carefully.

You can often purchase pre-cut fruit and vegetables in your produce section. Before you buy, check to see where they cut the fruit. You can get cross contamination is they used a shared counter.

Dairy Products

The majority of your dairy products are gluten free. Highly processed dairy products may not be, however, so check the ingredients listed.

Plain milk, heavy cream, butter and plain yogurt are gluten free. If you get a flavored yogurt, read the label.

Also avoid yogurt that comes with granola or cookies as they will contain gluten.

Most cheese is gluten free, just avoid beer washed cheeses and blue cheese. Sometimes a manufacturer will use wheat as a catalyst in the production of blue cheese. You may have to reach out to specific manufacturers to find one that does not do this. Be careful of cheese that is repackaged at the store. A lot of the stores will use the same surface for slicing cheese that they do slicing bread and making sandwiches which can lead to contamination.

As far as ice cream goes, always read your labels. You can automatically omit any flavors that have cookies, cookie dough, pretzels, graham cracker crust or any other name that would raise the gluten red flag.

Grains

Many grains, flours, bread, pasta and cereals are off limits, but you can still find some very good grain choices. Millet, hominy, flax and rice are great grains that are gluten free as long as they are not mixed with or processed with gluten containing grains, preservatives or additives.

Flours that are gluten free include rice, corn, bean, soy and potato. Tapioca also has the green light and arrowroot is a great gluten free thickening agent. Amaranth, buckwheat, corn, cornmeal, soy and sorghum are also OK. There is some controversy surrounding oats because of cross contamination. But you can always check with the manufacturer regarding how the oats are grown (if they are grown in the same field as wheat or harvested with equipment that also harvests wheat), processed (in the same plants as wheat) and packaged then make your own determination.

Quinoa is an absolutely awesome grain! Actually, it is a seed, but is used as a grain. You can have it in the morning with fresh fruit, mix it with fresh cucumber, onion and bell pepper for lunch, or create a savory side with dinner. It is very versatile and full of nutrients.

Always avoid wheat, farina, rye, semolina, triticale, graham flour, barley (malt vinegar, malt flavoring and malt are typically made from barley), bulgur, kamut and durum flour. These are wheat products and do contain gluten.

A word on canned and processed foods

Canned and processed foods are generally unhealthy

regardless of gluten content. They are typically loaded with sodium and various preservatives that you cannot even pronounce, much less want inside your body. From a gluten related standpoint, though, there is a great danger of cross contamination in the canning and preparation processes. If you must use canned and processed foods do so with extreme caution and read your labels carefully.

Pre-packaged foods

We live in a world of convenience and pre-packaged, processed foods are the staple of many American homes. Many of those processed foods, though are not only unhealthy, they contain gluten. These are some of the more common processed foods that you should avoid unless they are specifically labeled "gluten free."

- Breads
- Tortilla chips
- Cereals
- Self-basting poultry
- Potato chips
- Croutons
- Matzo
- Salad dressing
- Cakes
- Soups

- Soup bases
- French fries
- Candies
- Seasoned rice mixes
- Gravies
- Soy sauce
- Cookies
- Vegetables in sauce
- Processed lunch meat
- Crackers
- Prepared grains that may be gluten free in its natural form

Substitutions

Use

Rice or quinoa with spices

Instead of

Prepared/seasoned rice or quinoa blend

Use

Spaghetti Squash, quinoa, rice noodles or soba noodles

Instead of

Pasta

Use

Butter, mashed ripe avocado or coconut oil (if you are also going dairy free)

Instead of
Margarine

Use
Combine to make 1 cup of gluten free flour blend:

¼ C potato starch or cornstarch
¼ C tapioca flour (or starch)
½ C rice flour

Instead of
1 C all-purpose flour

Use
Cornstarch, egg or arrowroot powder
Instead of
Flour to thicken roux or gravy

Use
Oats (gluten free)

Instead of
Breadcrumbs

Use

Romaine lettuce leaves

Instead of

Sandwich or pita bread

Spices

Of course, the fat and spices are what bring out the flavor in your food. Spices should not be a concern in a gluten free diet. Pretty much all fresh herbs that you get in the produce section of your supermarket are fine. Most single ingredient dried spices are gluten free, but for blends you should read the label. It should not take you long to find the manufacturers that are conscientious and transparent with their customers.

Plain salt and pepper are gluten free, but flavored salts and peppers may not be. Read the labels or check with the manufacturer.

When purchasing extracts (vanilla, lemon, etc.) look for extracts made with an Ethyl Alcohol, not grain based alcohol. When in doubt, contact the manufacturer.

Many types of mustard are considered gluten free as are some ketchups. However, if you have trouble with gluten based vinegars you may have a problem with these condiments as most ketchups and mustards have them. Look for ingredients such as apple cider vinegar or rice vinegar instead.

If you like flavored oils (basil, garlic, etc.), your best bet is to do it yourself. Some store bought flavored oils are not gluten free.

Spice Staples

Sea Salt (fine)
Coarse Ground Black Pepper
Sweet Basil
Oregano
Paprika
Smoked Paprika
Parsley
Garlic Powder
Onion Powder

You might also want to keep some fresh ginger on hand. If you juice, drop a ½ to 1 inch piece in with the fruits you are juicing. It gives it a nice flavor. It is also nice with salads, in sauces for chicken and seafood and in dressings. Just remember to use a light hand. Ginger is very strong and it doesn't take much to get that boost of flavor.

7 Day Meal Plan with Menus

Try these gluten free meal plans incorporating the recipes contained within this book. Pair them with any of the dishes listed in the Vegetables and Side Dishes section of this book and you will have a well-rounded meal.

Sunday

Breakfast: Gluten Free Pancakes with Maple Syrup
Lunch: Chicken Wrap
Dinner: Hearty Beef Stew

Monday

Breakfast: Apple Blueberry Quinoa
Lunch: Honey Glazed Salmon over Greens
Dinner: Home style Burgers

Tuesday

Breakfast: Chicken Sausage and Cheese Quiche
Lunch: Buttermilk Ranch Chicken Green Salad
Dinner: Apricot Chicken

Wednesday

Breakfast: Oatmeal with Cinnamon, Brown Sugar Apples
Lunch: Roasted Vegetables Quinoa Salad
Dinner: Salmon Fajitas

Thursday

Breakfast: Chicken Mushroom and Brown Rice Frittata
Lunch: Chicken Burger
Dinner: Paprika Chicken

Friday

Breakfast: Banana Split Oatmeal
Lunch: Tuna Salad Wrap
Dinner: Cajun Jambalaya

Saturday

Breakfast: Cajun Egg Scramble
Lunch: Stuffed Zucchini
Dinner: Broccoli Cheddar Bake

Recipes

These are complete recipes for breakfast, lunch, dinner and snacks. You can mix and match to create delicious menus for weeks. Also, many of the recipes have options at the end for different, interesting variations. Gluten free does not have to be tasteless and boring!

The measurement abbreviations are as follows:

t = teaspoon
T = Tablespoon
C = Cup
Dash = About 1/8 teaspoon

Breakfast

Banana Split Oatmeal

This is always a favorite among young and old alike. It takes a favorite dessert and turns it into a delicious, healthy breakfast!

½ C Gluten Free Oatmeal
1 ¼ C Water
½ Small Banana, coarsely chopped
2 - 3 Large Strawberries, coarsely chopped
¼ C Semi-Sweet Chocolate Chips
Chopped Nuts (walnuts, pecans, hazelnuts)
Dash Salt

NOTE: This recipe "grows" so use a medium saucepan.

This makes one large serving, but you can easily double it to feed two or three people.

In medium saucepan, bring water to a boil. Stir in oatmeal. Add salt, banana and strawberry. Let cook for about 5 minutes, remove from heat.

Spoon oatmeal into a bowl and add chocolate chips and nuts. Enjoy!

You can top with a dollop of vanilla yogurt for a whipped cream effect.

Variations:

Use Kasha (toasted buckwheat) or Quinoa instead of Oatmeal

½ Small Apple, coarsely chopped (gala are super sweet, ambrosia are milder)

1 – 2 t Brown Sugar

Cinnamon to Taste

Add any berries (or combinations) including: blueberries, raspberries, blackberries

Honey with a dab of gluten free vanilla yogurt

Apple Blueberry Quinoa

Quinoa is such a wonderful, versatile food! It can go sweet or savory. Quinoa is actually a seed, but it is used as a grain making it a delicious, high protein, gluten free grain substitute!

1 C Quinoa
2 C Water
½ Small Apple
¼ C Fresh Blueberries
Cinnamon
Honey
Rinse quinoa.

In a medium saucepan, bring quinoa and water to a boil. Reduce heat to medium low and simmer for about 5 minutes.

Add apples, blueberries and cinnamon. Continue simmering until all of the water has been absorbed.

Spoon into a bowl and drizzle with honey.

NOTE: If you prefer your apples more cooked, include them when you first put the quinoa on to cook.

Variations:

You can also add or substitute dates, raisins, raspberries, bananas or chopped nuts
Top with vanilla yogurt, milk or vanilla almond milk
Add nutmeg, allspice or pumpkin pie spice

Gluten Free Pancakes with Maple Syrup

These awesome pancakes definitely do not taste gluten free! Pair them with a few pats of butter and real maple syrup and you have fantastic breakfast!

1 C Sour Cream
1C Ricotta Cheese
¾ C Gluten Free Flour (see recipe in "Substitutions")
4 Eggs, separated
2 T Honey
¾ t Salt
2 t Vanilla Extract
Cinnamon to Taste
Butter
Maple Syrup

Mix sour cream, ricotta, flour, egg yolks, honey, salt and vanilla. You may want to use a mixer, food processor or blender to get the ingredients well mixed.

In a large bowl, whisk the egg whites well (until stiff peaks begin to form), add the pancake batter into the bowl and fold the egg whites into the mixture.

Butter griddle or pan and cook pancakes over a medium low heat. You may flip them a couple of times to ensure they are a nice golden brown on both sides.

Serve with butter and real maple syrup.

Variations:

You may add blueberries, strawberries, chopped apples, banana, raspberries, chopped nuts or chocolate chips

Cajun Egg Scramble

This recipe is taken from the bayous of Louisiana and adapted to be gluten free. But it still keeps its Cajun flavor!

Cajun Shrimp
2 C Salad Shrimp
1 C Chopped Tomato
¼ C Chopped Sweet Onion
1 t Chopped Garlic
1 T Fresh Parsley
Sea Salt
Coarse Ground Black Pepper
Tabasco

Over medium heat cook shrimp, tomato, onion, garlic, parsley and seasonings in a little oil or butter until the shrimp and tomato are cooked. Set aside.

Scrambled Eggs
1 t Butter
6 Eggs
¼ C Milk
1 t Sweet Basil
Sea Salt
Coarse Ground Black Pepper

Beat all ingredients in a large bowl until eggs are well beaten. Add Cajun Shrimp to the egg mixture and beat well.

Melt butter in a large pan over medium heat. Pour egg mixture into the pan and cook. As egg cooks, use a rubber spatula to gently scrape the cooked eggs from the sides and bottom of the pan, moving it towards the center. Keep the mixture moving constantly to prevent scorching and to keep the egg somewhat separated.

Serve with gluten free tortillas or alone as a Cajun omelet.

Variations:

You can substitute the shrimp for chicken, gluten free chicken sausage or turkey

Oatmeal with Cinnamon-Brown Sugar-Maple Apples

Oatmeal has long been a breakfast staple. It is quick, easy and you can dress it up with just about anything you want. Apples really bring a lot to this dish. Try gala apples for extra sweetness, or ambrosia for a more subtle sweet.

½ C Gluten Free Oatmeal
1 ¼ C Water
½ Small Apple, coarsely chopped
1 t Brown Sugar (or to taste)
½ t Cinnamon (or to taste)

In medium saucepan, heat the water to boiling. Add apple, brown sugar and cinnamon. Reduce heat and cook until apple becomes soft, about 5 minutes. For softer apples, cook a little longer, but you may have to add more water when you cook your oatmeal.

When apples are almost cooked, add oatmeal, stir well and cook for 5 minutes or until oatmeal is cooked. Serve and enjoy.

Variations:

Add any berries, nuts, banana/walnut, sweet potato, pumpkin/pecan

Stir in cream, milk or vanilla yogurt for a creamier consistency

Chicken, Mushroom and Brown Rice Frittata

You can't hardly go wrong with a frittata! You throw some stuff together and you have a great meal. This frittata is a great breakfast, but it would make a wonderful brunch as well.

½ C Brown Rice
2 C Water
2 Chicken Breasts, chopped
½ Small Sweet Onion, chopped
½ - 1 Pound Fresh Mushrooms, chopped
½ Green Bell Pepper, chopped (you can add some red bell pepper too for more color)
1 T Garlic, minced
6 Large Eggs
2 T milk
2 T Fresh Parsley, chopped
2 T Fresh Basil, chopped
Sea Salt
Coarse Ground Black Pepper
½ C Shredded Cheese Blend Parmesan and Mozzarella

Prepare rice with water and a dash of salt in a small saucepan. Bring to a boil, then reduce heat to a simmer, cover and cook for about 40 minutes (until rice is tender). Once cooked, you should have 1 ½ C rice.

While rice is cooking, in an ovenproof skillet, add a little oil and cook the chicken, onion, mushroom, garlic and bell pepper, as well as a little salt and pepper, until chicken is cooked through. Stir in the rice, Set aside.

Beat the eggs, milk, parsley, basil, salt and pepper in a large bowl.

Place the rack in your oven in the upper third section and preheat the broiler.

Pour the egg mixture over the rice, meat and vegetable mixture (in the ovenproof skillet). Cook on medium low heat, partially covered, for about 5 minutes (until eggs start to pull away from the sides of the pan). Remove from heat.

Sprinkle the cheese over the frittata and place pan (uncovered) in the oven. Cook under the broiler for about 2 minutes. Eggs will be set and cheese on top will be browned.

Let stand about 5 minutes. Serve.

Variations:

Instead of Chicken add gluten free chicken sausage, beef, turkey

Omit the meat and add more veggies such as tomato, fresh spinach, zucchini and squash

Sprinkle toasted flax seed over the top for a nutty flavor and fiber boost

Chicken Sausage and Cheese Quiche

Quiches are marvelous dishes. You can just grab whatever is in the fridge, toss it in and voila! You have breakfast (or brunch)! Make sure you check out the variations section at the end of this recipe for some great dish versatility.

24 Ounces Frozen Hash Browns (plain or flavored), thawed
½ C Melted Butter
1 C Gluten Free Chicken Sausage, chopped and cooked
1 C Colby Jack Cheese, shredded
2 Eggs
1 t Sweet Basil
Salt
Coarse Ground Black Pepper
½ C Heavy Whipping Cream
Preheat oven to 425 Degrees F.

Blot potatoes on paper towels to remove excess moisture.

In a bowl, combine potatoes and butter. Press mixture into the bottom and sides of an ungreased pie pan.

Bake your "crust" at 425 degrees for about 25 minutes.

Remove from oven and add the chicken sausage and half of the cheese to cover the bottom of the "crust."
In a separate bowl, beat the eggs, basil, salt, pepper and cream. Pour mixture over the chicken sausage and cheese.

Sprinkle top with remaining cheese.

Return to oven and bake at 425 degrees for about 30 minutes or until eggs are completely set.

Variations:

Try the flavored hash browns such as garlic and herb. Just read the label to make sure they are gluten free.

Add a little onion or garlic to the melted butter before you mix it with the hash browns.

Substitute the chicken sausage for seasoned beef, turkey or even shrimp or salmon.

Lunch

Honey Ginger Glazed Salmon over Greens

Honey glazed salmon is a favorite dish with a lot of people. Pair it with a nice bed of greens and you have a healthy, delicious salad that will give you a nice boost of Omega 3's.

Salmon

2 Salmon Filets
1 T Grape Seed Oil or Extra Virgin Olive Oil
2 t Honey (clover or wildflower are best)
1 t Smoked Paprika
1 t Basil
1 t Garlic, minced
¼ t Fresh Ginger, grated
¼ t Red Pepper Flakes, crushed (may add more or less to taste)
Salt
Coarse Ground Black Pepper
Fresh Lemon

Salad

1 C Fresh Romaine Lettuce, cut

1 C Fresh Baby Spinach

¼ C Red Cabbage, shredded

½ C Carrots, shredded

¼ C Sweet Onion, sliced

Dressing

¼ C Grape Seed Oil (see Variations below for more oil options)

2 T Apple Cider Vinegar

1 ½ t Shallots, finely chopped

1 t Dijon Mustard (plain or honey)

Heat oven to 325 degrees F. Place oven rack to the middle position.

In a bowl, combine the oil, honey, paprika, basil, garlic, ginger, pepper flakes, salt and black pepper. Whisk until completely blended. Chill in the refrigerator for 20 to 39 minutes to allow flavors to blend.

In another bowl or bottle, combine the oil, apple cider vinegar, shallots and mustard. Mix well and refrigerate until ready to use.

Pat salmon dry then spritz with fresh lemon juice (just a touch). Very lightly coat with a little oil (or melted butter) and place in an oven proof dish.

Remove glaze mixture from the refrigerator and very gently whisk it a couple of times to distribute the garlic and shallots throughout the glaze. Pour over the salmon filets.

Bake at 325 degrees for 20 to 25 minutes or until the fish flakes easily with a fork.

Cut the salmon into pieces.

Assemble the salad by combining all of the ingredients in a large bowl. Add the salmon and drizzle with the dressing.

Top with pecans, walnuts, sunflower seeds or other favorite salad toppers.

Variations:

Oil – Extra Virgin Olive Oil has a heavier, earthy flavor, Sesame Oil has a nutty flavor, Avocado Oil has an almost buttery flavor

Substitute chicken or turkey for the salmon.

Toss in cooked shrimp.

Chicken Wrap

This is an extremely versatile dish but what's more, it is a wrap with a twist. Instead of using traditional tortillas as wraps, this recipe uses romaine lettuce leaves. What a neat, no carb and gluten free idea!

2 – 3 Large Romaine Lettuce Leaves, rinsed and patted dry
2 Chicken Breasts, boneless, skinless, cut into strips, cooked
1 Small Cucumber, peeled and cut into strips
½ Avocado, peeled and cut into strips
1 Roma Tomato, cut into strips
¼ Small Sweet Onion, thinly sliced
1 t Toasted Flax Seeds
2 T Pecans, chopped
Salt
Coarse Ground Black Pepper

Lay the Romaine lettuce leaves on a plate. Lay the chicken strips, cucumber, avocado, tomato and onion on the lettuce, leaving one edge free to wrap.

Sprinkle the flax seeds and pecans over the chicken and vegetables. Salt and pepper to taste.

Fold the free edge of the lettuce over the chicken and vegetables to form a wrap.

NOTE:

When you only use half of an avocado, leave the pit in the half you are storing and it will not turn brown. Just place that half with the pit in a storage bag or container and refrigerate.

Variations:

Use shrimp, salmon, turkey or beef instead of chicken.

Drizzle with your favorite gluten free salad dressing to dress your wrap up a bit.

Add red pepper flakes for a little heat.

Buttermilk Ranch Chicken Green Salad

Buttermilk ranch dressing is very popular on salads and even sandwiches but when you pair this homemade buttermilk ranch dressing with chicken and a green salad, WOW.

2 Chicken Breasts, chopped into bite sized pieces
1 C Fresh Baby Spinach
1 C Fresh Romaine Lettuce, chopped
1 C Fresh Mushrooms, chopped (button mushrooms are best for this)
½ C Carrots, shredded
½ C Red Cabbage, shredded
½ Green Bell Pepper, sliced (you can add red and yellow peppers as well)
2 Roma Tomatoes, chopped
½ Sweet Onion, sliced in wedges
2 Boiled Eggs, chopped
Shredded Cheese (Colby Jack or Mild Cheddar)
Salt
Coarse Ground Black Pepper

Dressing

1 C Buttermilk
½ C Mayonnaise (NOT salad dressing!)

1 t Apple Cider Vinegar

1 T Fresh Parsley

1 T Fresh Basil

1 t Fresh Chives, finely chopped

¼ t Mustard Powder

¼ t Black Pepper

¼ t Paprika

1/8 t Dill

In a medium bowl, combine the mayonnaise and buttermilk. Whisk thoroughly until they are completely blended. Add the remaining ingredients, whisk till blended.

Put in a bottle or container and refrigerate for at least 30 minutes before serving.

Season the chicken with salt and pepper. Cook in a medium pan over medium heat until done.

In a large bowl, combine the spinach, lettuce, mushrooms, carrots, cabbage, bell pepper, tomato and onion. Sprinkle a little salt and pepper then toss lightly.

Top with egg, cheese and cooked chicken. Serve with salad dressing.

Variations:

Toss in whatever vegetables are in season such as squash, zucchini, radishes, etc.

Substitute the apple cider vinegar in the dressing for lemon juice.

Add a little red pepper flakes or cayenne pepper to the chicken or salad dressing for a kick of heat.

Stuffed Zucchini

This is a pretty simple dish with a lot of flavor. It is filling and will soon become a favorite in your home. The stuffing is absolutely irresistible!

4 Medium Zucchini, cut in half long ways
1 pound Ground Chicken
12 oz. or 1 pound Gluten Free Chicken Sausage, chopped
1 Small Sweet Onion, chopped
2 t Garlic, minced
½ C Brown Rice, cooked
1 Egg, beaten with a splash of milk or cream
1 can Crushed Tomatoes
½ t Sugar
1 C Gluten Free Chicken Stock
Fresh Mozzarella Cheese, shredded
Salt
Coarse Ground Black Pepper

Preheat oven to 350 degrees F. Spray a 13X9 inch baking dish (use a deep dish such as a cake pan).

Use a spoon to scoop out the seeds from the zucchini. Save about ½ to ¾ of them to put in your stuffing.

In a medium bowl, combine the chicken, chicken

sausage, onion, garlic, rice, egg and zucchini seeds. Season with a dash of salt and pepper (don't overdo it with the salt, the chicken stock will provide ample salt).

Pile meat mixture in the zucchini halves (it should be piled high).

Combine the tomatoes (with the juice), sugar and chicken stock. Mix well and liberally spoon over the meat stuffing in the zucchini halves.

Place in oven and bake at 350 degrees for 40 minutes. Remove from the oven and top with cheese. Return to oven and bake for an additional 5 minutes or until cheese is melted. Depending on the oven, it may take a little longer to cook. Check and make sure the chicken is fully cooked before serving.

NOTE:

You may want to put a cookie sheet or foil under the pan while baking because this dish bubbles and splatters quite a bit.

Variations:

Substitute the brown rice for cooked quinoa

Substitute the crushed tomatoes for Rotel™ Tomatoes for a little spice
Instead of the chicken sausage, use chopped, cooked shrimp.

Tuna Salad Wrap

With romaine lettuce leaves as the wrap, this good old standby gets a little face lift. Check out the variations of this recipe as well. You can go classic or fancy.

Several Large Leaves of Romaine Lettuce, rinsed and patted dry
1 can Tuna Packed in Water, rinsed and drained
2 -3 T Mayonnaise
2 -3 Boiled Eggs, chopped
¼ Sweet Onion, chopped
1 T Sweet Pickle Relish
½ - 1 t Dijon Mustard

Combine tuna, mayonnaise, egg, onion, pickle relish and mustard in a medium bowl.

Use 2 or 3 Romaine leaves as a wrap. Place some tuna salad on the leaves and roll it as a wrap.

Variations:

Substitute Dijon mustard for honey Dijon mustard.

Substitute cream cheese or sour cream instead of all or part of the mayonnaise.

Add chopped tomato, bell pepper, celery or cucumber to the salad.

Roasted Vegetables Quinoa Salad

There is just something about roasted vegetables that is so comforting. Combine it with quinoa and it is just heavenly. This could be the new, gluten free comfort food!

1 – 2 C Quinoa, cooked
Roasted Vegetables
1 C Sugar Snap Peas
1 C Baby Carrots
½ Green Bell Pepper, cut in bite sized chunks
½ Red Bell Pepper, cut into bite sized chunks
1 Medium Tomato, chopped
1 Yellow Squash, chopped
1 Zucchini, chopped
1 C Mushrooms, chopped
2 T Garlic, minced
1 C Nuts (walnuts, pecans, almonds, pine nuts, hazelnuts), chopped
2 T Extra Virgin Olive Oil or Grape Seed Oil
3 T Parmesan Cheese, shredded
3 t Sweet Basil
3 t Garlic Powder
3 t Parsley
Salt
Coarse Ground Black Pepper

Heat oven to 400 degrees F.

In a large bowl, combine all vegetables. Drizzle with oil and add spices and cheese. Mix thoroughly. Place in a foil lined baking pan and bake at 400 degrees for 45 minutes or until vegetables are soft and roasted.

When done, add vegetables to quinoa. Top with nuts and sprinkle cheese over the top.

Variations:

For a nutty flavor, use sesame seed oil instead of olive oil.

Add nuts to the vegetables so that they cook together.

Use whole or halved garlic cloves instead of minced garlic.

Add a little zing by combining 2 T apple cider vinegar, 2 T extra virgin olive oil, ¼ t ginger, dash salt and coarse ground black pepper. If you are feeling particularly feisty add a little cayenne. Mix well and refrigerate 30 minutes before using.

Chicken Burger

An ordinary chicken burger that is anything but ordinary! One bite of this baby and you will be hooked!

1 pound Ground Chicken
½ C Brown Rice, cooked
½ Sweet Onion, chopped
½ t Worcestershire Sauce
½ t Garlic Powder
½ t Onion Powder
Salt
Coarse Ground Black Pepper

In a large bowl, combine all ingredients. Mix well so that seasoning is evenly distributed.

Use a large serving spoon to measure the meat for the patties. Using your hands, form them into balls then flatten them to 1 inch thick or less.

Heat a pan with oil over medium heat. You will need to keep the pan moist as ground chicken has very little fat. Cook evenly, flipping at least once (about 4 minutes on one side, then about 3 minutes on the other side).

Serve on gluten free buns or on a bed of lettuce.

NOTE:

Ground chicken is very mild so you don't need a lot of spice to season it.

Ground chicken also cooks fairly quickly so you need to stay near it while it is cooking.

Variations:

You can use ground turkey instead of chicken.

You can also use chopped mushrooms or cooked quinoa instead of the rice to hold the patties together.

Add chopped tomatoes, mild nuts or seeds or chopped zucchini to your meat mixture.

Chop shrimp, season well and mix in with the ground meat.

Dinner

Apricot Chicken

This dish tastes like something you would get in a restaurant but it is so stinking easy to make! The flavors blend to create a dish that is absolute perfection. This will quickly become a favorite in your house!

2 Boneless Skinless Chicken Breasts
½ C Apricot Preserves
1 T Soy Sauce (gluten free)
1 T Brown Sugar
Oil
Salt
Pepper

Using a mallet, pound chicken breasts until thin, about ½ to 1 inch; salt and pepper to taste. Heat some oil in a pan over medium heat. Add chicken breasts and cook until brown and almost cooked through.

Remove breasts from pan and add apricot preserves, soy sauce and brown sugar (you may want to adjust the brown sugar up or down according to taste). Stir constantly until mixture is bubbling. Return breasts to pan, spoon apricot mixture over breasts, reduce heat, cover and simmer for 3 to 4 minutes. Stir sauce occasionally and watch your heat so it does not scorch.

Flip breasts and cook another 3 to 4 minutes. Remove from heat. Spoon warm apricot glaze over breasts before serving.

Variations:

Use salmon or shrimp instead of chicken.

Use raspberry preserves and a splash of heavy cream instead of apricot preserves and soy sauce.

Cajun Jambalaya

Another authentic Cajun staple brought to your table. This is so easy to make with simple ingredients. Now you can get a taste of Louisiana anytime you want!

6 or 8 Chicken Thighs, skinned, deboned and cut into bite sized pieces
1 C Gluten Free Chicken Sausage, chopped or sliced
1 Medium Sweet Onion, chopped
2 T Garlic, minced
1 – 2 Stalks Celery, chipped
1 Green Bell Pepper, Chopped (add red and/or yellow for another layer of flavor and more color)
3 C Rice (uncooked – white or brown)
4 C Water
Butter
Cajun Spice
1 T Garlic Powder
1 T Onion Powder
3 t Paprika
1 t Oregano
2 t Brown Sugar
½ - 1 t Cayenne Pepper
Salt
Coarse Ground Black Pepper

In a large saucepan or Dutch oven over medium high heat, melt 3 to 4 tablespoons of butter. Generously season the chicken with Cajun seasoning then place chicken and vegetables in the saucepan with the butter. Sauté chicken and vegetables for about 5 minutes, add the gluten free chicken sausage and cook another 5 minutes.

Add water, scraping the bottom of the pan to loosen any chicken or seasoning. Add the rice, stir well and bring to a boil.

Reduce heat to a simmer, cover and cook until the rice is completely cooked, about 30 – 45 minutes). Watch closely and do not allow the bottom to scorch. You may have to reduce the heat further.

Variations:

Substitute the chicken for shrimp, (real) crab, salmon.

Substitute the gluten free chicken sausage for highly seasoned shrimp.

Add some Rotel® Tomatoes for a spicy kick.

Chicken Broccoli Cheddar Bake

This is an updated version of an old classic. Cheddar and broccoli blend together with brown rice to create a filling, very satisfying meal.

1 Package (16 oz.) Broccoli, chopped, thawed
2 C Brown Rice, cooked
½ Sweet Onion, chopped
2 t Garlic, minced
5 Eggs, lightly beaten with about 1 teaspoon of cream
1 C Milk
½ C Chicken Stock
1 ½ C Mild Cheddar Cheese, shredded
½ C Mild Cheddar Cheese, shredded
Garlic Powder
Salt
Coarse Ground Black Pepper
Preheat oven to 350 degrees F.

In a large bowl, combine the broccoli, rice, onion, garlic, eggs, milk, chicken stock and the 1 ½ cups cheddar cheese. Season with the garlic powder, salt and pepper to taste.

Pour into a greased casserole dish and sprinkle the remaining ½ cup cheddar cheese over the top.

Bake at 350 degrees for 1 hour (until top is lightly brown and set).

Variations:

Use 1 cup mild cheddar and 1 cup medium or sharp cheddar instead of mild cheddar only.

Use other vegetables such as asparagus, zucchini, squash and tomatoes, either combined or separately instead of or with the broccoli.

Toss in some cooked chicken, beef or shrimp for an extra kick of protein.

Home style Burgers

Sometimes you just want a good home made burger. Well, this is definitely the recipe! You can also have some fun trying the different variations.

1 pound Lean Ground Beef
½ Sweet Onion, chopped
2 t Garlic, minced
1 T Worcestershire Sauce
Garlic Powder
Salt
Coarse Ground Black Pepper

Mix all ingredients together and let sit in the refrigerator for about 30 minutes.

Heat a little oil in a pan over medium heat. Form patties with the meat mixture and place them in the pan. Cover and let cook for 4 – 5 minutes. Flip and let cook for another 3 – 4 minutes for medium burgers. Cook a little longer for well-done burgers.

Serve alone with some barbeque sauce or ketchup, or serve on gluten free buns with all the trimmings.

NOTE:

You can tell how done your burger is by pressing on it in the middle. First, gently press the center of your chin, right at the end of the chin bone. That degree of cushion is what a medium rare burger will feel like. If you press the area between your eyes, that is how a medium well burger will feel. Use that as a gauge to determine the doneness of your burger.

Variations:

Use ground turkey instead of beef or use half ground turkey and half beef.

When you form your patties, put a slice of cheese inside the middle of the patty.

Chop some cooked, seasoned shrimp and mix it in with your ground meat for another layer of flavor; a real taste adventure!

Hearty Beef Stew

The ultimate in comfort food, beef stew has everything you need for a meal in one pot. Toss in whatever vegetables are in season and enjoy!

1 pound Beef, cut into bite sized pieces (any cut is good for beef stew)
3 T Extra Virgin Olive Oil
1 Sweet Onion, chopped
1 Green Bell Pepper, chopped
1 pound Mushrooms, chopped
2 stalks Celery, chopped
2 – 3 C Beef Stock
2 T + 2 t Arrowroot Powder
3 t Garlic, minced
2 large Potatoes, washed and cut into bite sized pieces
1 C Baby Carrots
1 C Fresh Green Beans
1 can Rotel™ Tomatoes or Crushed Tomatoes
1 T Worcestershire Sauce
1 t Rosemary, dried and crushed
1 t Thyme, dried
Salt
Coarse Ground Black Pepper

In a large pot, heat the oil over a medium high flame.

Season the meat well with salt, pepper and Worcestershire Sauce. Once the oil is very hot (when it starts to smoke a little) add the beef and brown it thoroughly.

Once the meat is browned, removed it from the pan with a slotted spoon (you want to leave the meat juices in the pan) and set it aside.

Add the onion, bell pepper, mushrooms and celery. Sauté until the onion is soft and almost transparent.

Reduce the heat to medium low. Add the arrowroot and cook for about 2 minutes, stirring often. If you need a little more oil, use just a bit. Add the garlic and cook for another minute or so.

Add about ¼ cup of the beef stock to the pan and deglaze, scraping up any of the brown bits that are stuck to the bottom of the pan and incorporating them into the gravy. You will see the gravy begin to thicken. Bring this mixture to a simmer for about 5 minutes.

Add the remaining broth, spices and meat. Cover and simmer on a low heat for about an hour.

Add the potatoes and carrots. Cook covered for an additional 30 minutes or until the vegetables are soft.

Remove from heat and allow to sit for about 20 minutes before serving.

Variation:

Put everything except for the arrowroot in a crockpot. Cook on high for 3 or 4 hours. Remove about ¼ to ½ cup of the broth. Put the arrowroot in a pan with some of the broth and cook, stirring constantly. Gradually add the remaining broth and cook until it begins to thicken. Return thickened gravy base to your crockpot and stir.

Paprika Chicken

This is another quick, easy dish that taste like it took you hours to make. The paprika gives such a sweet, mild flavor to the chicken and the onions and mushrooms really set it off. Very pretty dish too.

2 Chicken Breasts, boneless, skinless
2 T Extra Virgin Olive Oil
1 Sweet Onion, sliced
½ pound Mushrooms, sliced
Paprika
Salt
Coarse Ground Black Pepper

Pound the chicken breasts with a mallet until they are very thin. Season generously with paprika, salt and pepper.

Heat oil in a pan over medium high flame. Toss the mushrooms in the pan for about 5 minutes.

Place the chicken in the pan and arrange the onion and mushrooms over and around the chicken. Sprinkle a little paprika, salt and pepper over the onion and mushrooms.

Cover and cook for 4 minutes.

If necessary, reduce heat to medium. Turn breasts over and move onions and mushrooms around in the pan so that the chicken can come in contact with the surface (at least part of the surface of the chicken should come in contact with the surface of the pan). Arrange some of the onion and mushrooms over the chicken breasts. Cook an additional 3 or 4 minutes.

Serve alone with the onion and mushrooms or over a bed of rice.

Salmon Fajitas

It's salmon and its fajitas, what a combination! Make your own gluten free tortillas and put this spicy little number together for a little trip south of the border!

Tortilla

2 C Gluten Free Flour (see recipe in "Substitutions")
2 t Guar Gum or Xanthan Gum
1 t Gluten Free Baking Powder
1 t salt
2 t Brown Sugar
1 C Warm Water
Extra Virgin Olive Oil
Salmon Filling
¼ C Extra Virgin Olive Oil
½ t Lime Zest
1 T Chili Powder
1 t Oregano
½ t Cumin, ground
Salt
Coarse Ground Black Pepper
3 T Extra Virgin Olive Oil
1 pound Salmon Filet, cut into chunks
1 medium Sweet Onion, sliced
½ Green Bell Pepper, sliced

½ Red Bell Pepper, sliced
Fresh Lime

To make the tortillas:

In a large mixing bowl, combine all dry ingredients thoroughly.

Add the warm water to the dry ingredients. Use your hands to mix so that it forms a moist dough.

Separate the dough into 8 balls. Keep all the dough balls covered in the bowl until you are ready to cook them.

Heat a griddle or large pan over medium heat. Pour a little oil in the pan and allow it to warm.

Taking one dough ball at a time, sprinkle some gluten free flour on a flat surface. Lightly dust your rolling pin as well. Place the dough ball on the floured surface and roll with the rolling pin until it is as thin as possible.

Place the rolled out tortilla on the hot pan and cook for about 2 minutes (It will start puffing up and there will be griddle marks on the underside of the tortilla). Flip the tortilla and cook for an additional 1 – 2 minutes (it will brown as well).

Put the tortilla on a covered plate so that it will stay warm.

Repeat with all of the dough balls until you have 8 cooked tortillas.

Cook the Salmon Filling:

In a small bowl, combine the ¼ cup oil and all spices including the lime zest.

Cover the bottom of a baking pan with the salmon chunks. Cover with the spice mixture. Refrigerate for about 30 minutes. (this is a good time to make your tortillas so they will be warm when your salmon is cooked)
In a medium pan, cook the onion and peppers in oil until onions begin to caramelize (about 15 minutes).

While onion and peppers are cooking, Place the salmon in a separate pan and cook over medium high heat (about 3 – 5 minutes).

To serve, place some salmon, onion and peppers on a tortilla and squeeze a little lime over it. Wrap and eat!

Vegetables and Sides

Steamed Broccoli

Steamed broccoli is a favorite in many restaurants, but when you prepare it this way you put even the best restaurants to shame! Toss in a little onion, a few mushrooms, yum!

1 pound Fresh Broccoli Crowns
4 – 6 Mushrooms, sliced
½ small Sweet Onion, sliced
Salt
Coarse Ground Black Pepper
1 t Garlic, minced
2 T Butter, softened

In a steamer or pot with a steam basket, arrange your broccoli, mushrooms and onion to cover the bottom of the basked evenly. Lightly season with salt and pepper.

Stir the garlic into the butter. Drop small dollops over the vegetables to cover evenly.

Cover pot and steam for 7 – 10 minutes or until broccoli turns a bright, brilliant green. Remove from steamer immediately and serve.

Cornbread Stuffing

This is another Louisiana recipe. It was originally written as an oyster stuffing. Now that variation is listed below the recipe – and you should try it! Unbelievably good!

Cornbread
4 T Butter, softened
1 T Sugar
2 Eggs, beaten slightly
½ C Milk
½ C Sour Cream
1 C Gluten Free Flour (see recipe in "Substitutions")
2 t Gluten Free Baking Powder
2/3 C Yellow Cornmeal
½ t Salt
Dressing
4 – 6 Chicken Thighs
4 Chicken Livers
2 C Gluten Free Cornbread (see recipe above)
2 C Gluten Free Bread Crumbs (you can substitute with 2 – 3 C Brown Rice if you prefer)
½ C Butter, cut into small pieces
6 – 8 Fresh Mushrooms, chopped
2 Green Onions, chopped (whites and tops)
1 C Chicken Stock
1 medium Sweet Onion, chopped

2 stalks Celery, chopped

1 raw Egg

2 boiled Eggs

Salt

Coarse Ground Black Pepper

Garlic Powder

Make Cornbread

Heat oven to 425 degrees F.

In a large bowl, combine butter and sugar. Beat until creamy. Mix eggs thoroughly into the butter. Add sour cream and milk. Make sure it is all mixed very well.

Add remaining dry ingredients and mix just until moist. Do not over mix.

Pour the cornbread batter into a greased pan and bake at 425 for about 20 minutes. You will know it is done when the top is golden brown and a toothpick inserted in the middle comes out clean.

Dressing

In a large pot, add onions and celery with a little chicken stock. Bring to a boil. Add the chicken thighs and make sure you have enough stock to cover then. Cover the pot and cook until the chicken is done. Add the chopped chicken liver to the pot when the chicken is done. Cook for about 4 or 5 minutes.

Remove chicken from the stock (save the stock!) and allow to cool. Debone and chop chicken.

While chicken is cooking, crumble the cornbread and gluten free white bread into a roaster or large baking pan. Sprinkle with some salt, pepper and garlic powder.

Add chicken to the bread mixture and slowly add the chicken stock with the onion and celery until the bread is moist.

Add the raw egg, mushroom, butter, boiled egg and green onion tops. Mix well.

Bake covered for about 30 minutes at 350 degrees. Uncover and bake an additional 30 – 45 minutes. You don't want to over brown it but you do want it to hold together.

Variations:

Add oysters to the chicken mixture. After the chicken has cooked, add the oysters and bring it to a boil.

Rice Pilaf

A pretty rice pilaf makes a nice compliment to just about any dish. Pair it with salmon or chicken. You will find it to have a mild flavor, yet it is quite satisfying.

2 C Brown Rice
4 C Chicken Stock
½ Sweet Onion, chopped
2 t Garlic, minced
½ - 1 C Sweet Peas, frozen
Place all ingredients into a large saucepan and bring to a boil. Reduce heat to medium low, cover and simmer until all moisture has been absorbed by rice and rice is done.

Serve and enjoy.

Potato Salad

You can't go to a barbeque or family picnic without this picnic standard. A little kick of apple cider vinegar gives it an interesting level of flavor that will make this your go to potato salad recipe!

2 pounds, Potatoes, peeled whole
1 ½ C Mayonnaise
1 T Apple Cider Vinegar
1 T Dijon Mustard
1 medium Sweet Onion, chopped
2 Celery Stalks, chopped
4 Hard Boiled Eggs, chopped
Salt
Course Ground Black Pepper

Place potatoes into a pot, add water so that they are just covered. Salt water and bring to a boil. Reduce heat to medium or medium high and cook for 30 – 35 minutes or until potatoes are tender (but not mushy). Drain and cut into cubes.

In a large bowl, combine mayonnaise, vinegar, mustard, salt and pepper. Add the celery, onion and potato chunks. Toss lightly. Gently stir in eggs.

Cover and refrigerate for 4 – 5 hours before serving.

Butter Herb Green Beans and New Potatoes

Herb butter lightly coats fresh green beans and new potatoes. Pair this side with any of the dishes on here and you will not be disappointed!

1 T Extra Virgin Olive Oil
1 ½ C New Potatoes, halved
1 ¼ Fresh Green Beans, snapped and trimmed
½ small Sweet Onion, sliced
¼ C Chicken Stock
Salt
Coarse Ground Black Pepper
1 t Rosemary, crushed
2 t Sweet Basil
1 t Garlic, minced
4 T Butter, melted

In a large pan, heat oil over medium high heat. Add potato, onion and beans. Salt and pepper lightly. Sauté for 3 minutes. Add ¼ chicken stock, cover and cook for 8 - 10 minutes or until beans are tender-crisp and potatoes are softened.

Remove potato and beans from the pan and place in a large, covered bowl.

In a small bowl, combine the melted butter, garlic, rosemary and basil. Mix well and drizzle over the potatoes and beans. Toss lightly to cover.

Steamed Asparagus with Garlic Butter

1 bunch Fresh Asparagus
2 t Garlic, minced
1 t Parsley
¼ C Butter

Rinse asparagus under cold water. Gently bend each stalk to find the natural break so you can remove the tough lower part of the stalk. Snap off the lower fibrous, tough part and retain the tender top part of the stalk.

In a steamer or pot with a steaming basket, heat the water and arrange the asparagus evenly across the basket. Cover and steam for 5 – 7 minutes (asparagus will get bright green).

In a small saucepan, melt the butter. Add the garlic and parsley. Keep warm until asparagus is cooked.

When done, remove asparagus from the steamer or pot and place in a wide dish that allows the stalks to be laid in a single or double layer over the bottom. Drizzle the herbed butter over the asparagus.

Serve warm.

Roasted Vegetables

This recipe will quickly become a family favorite. As the vegetables roast, the flavors blend with just the right amount of spices. You will find yourself eating this right out of the pan!

2 Fresh Yellow Squash, chopped
2 Fresh Zucchini, chopped
1 Sweet Onion, chopped
2 medium Tomatoes, chopped
2 C Fresh Mushrooms, chopped
1 C Baby Carrots
1 C Fresh Broccoli Crowns
6 – 8 Garlic Cloves, split
¼ - ½ C Sesame Seed Oil
Salt
Coarse Ground Black Pepper
Sweet Basil
Smoked Paprika
¼ C Parmesan Cheese, shredded
Heat oven to 350 degrees.

In large bowl, combine all vegetables. Add oil. Generously season with salt, pepper and basil. Add just a hint of smoked paprika (about 1 t). Mix well. Add the Parmesan cheese.

Place vegetables into a foil lined baking pan and spread evenly. You can sprinkle with a little more cheese and paprika. Cover and bake for 45 minutes. Uncover, switch oven to broil and cook an additional 15 – 20 minutes or until vegetables are browned on top and juice is bubbly.

Variations:

If you don't like the nuttiness of the sesame seed oil, use extra virgin olive oil instead.

Add or omit any vegetables that you wish.

This is great tossed on a green salad, combined with chicken or fish, tossed in cooked quinoa or eaten alone.

Creamy Tomato Soup

Served warm or cold, this creamy tomato soup has several varieties of tomatoes, roasted to perfection and blended with perfectly complimentary spices.

Assortment of Tomatoes (about 4 – 6), cut in half
4 Cherry Tomatoes, whole
½ Sweet Onion, sliced
6 cloves Garlic, peeled
Extra Virgin Olive Oil
2 C Chicken Stock
Butter
Salt
Coarse Ground Black Pepper
4 Fresh Basil Leaves
2 Bay Leaves

Preheat oven to 450 degrees F.

Arrange tomatoes, whole cherry tomatoes, onion and garlic on a baking sheet. Drizzle with olive oil and sprinkle with salt and pepper.

Roast vegetables in the oven for 25 – 30 minutes.

Remove vegetables from the oven and place in a stock

pot with the chicken stock. Add 2 – 4 tablespoons of butter and bay leaves. Bring to a boil then reduce heat and simmer for 15 – 20 minutes.

Remove bay leaves and process the tomato mixture with the basil in a blender or food processor in batches until smooth.

Season with a pinch of sugar, salt and pepper. Add some cayenne for a little fire. Drizzle with cream and sprinkle some fresh basil on top.

Snacks

Spicy Nut Mix

Keep this in your briefcase or bag so that you can get a little boost when your energy wanes. Go spicy or not, that's your choice. Experiment with your favorite spices and create your own mix!

½ C Natural Almonds
½ C Natural Walnuts
½ C Natural Pecans
½ C Natural Peanuts
Coarse Sea Salt
Coarse Ground Black Pepper
Red Pepper Flakes, crushed
2 T Extra Virgin Olive Oil

Place nuts in a bowl, drizzle with olive oil and add seasoning to taste. Toss lightly to coat.

To enhance the flavors, spread seasoned nuts on a cookie sheet and toast in a 250 degree oven for 10 – 15 minutes.

Bean Dip with Kale Chips

This bean dip is also great with gluten free chips and crackers, but the kale chips are actually quite good. Spritz with lemon before adding seasoning and cooking to alleviate some of the bitterness of the kale.

Bean Dip
2 C Red Beans
4 C Chicken Stock
1 T Worcestershire Sauce
2 t Garlic, minced
½ small Sweet Onion, minced
2 T Sour Cream
Salt
Coarse Ground Black Pepper
Cook red beans in chicken stock with Worcestershire sauce, garlic and onion. Season to taste.

When beans are done, place in a blender or food processor, with the sour cream and blend until smooth.

Kale Chips
1 bunch Fresh Kale
Extra Virgin Olive Oil
Garlic Powder
Salt

Coarse Ground Black Pepper

Preheat oven to 350 degrees F.

Line a cookie sheet with parchment paper.

Use a knife or kitchen shears to remove the leaves of the kale from the stems. Wash thoroughly and dry very well. Tear the leaves into bite sized pieces.

Arrange the kale on the cookie sheet and drizzle with oil. Sprinkle with seasoning. Bake for 10 – 15 minutes until edges are slightly brown but not burnt.

Tomato Basil Veggie Dip

This is much like your basic pesto, but with a dash of roasted tomato. The result is a fantastic dip for veggies or a nice condiment for chicken or shrimp. Keep some in your fridge and experiment. The possibilities are endless!

1 Roma Tomato, sliced
½ C Fresh Basil
¼ C Pine Nuts
2 cloves Garlic
½ C Extra Virgin Olive Oil
¼ C Parmesan Cheese, shredded
Salt
Coarse Ground Black Pepper

Heat oven to 400 degrees F.

Place tomato slices on a cookie sheet, drizzle with oil and sprinkle with salt and pepper.

Put tomato in the oven and roast for 15 – 20 minutes or until tomato is cooked.

Add roasted tomato, basil, pine nuts and garlic in a food processor. Add a little of the oil and blend well. Slowly add the oil as you blend and puree the vegetables. Taste and add salt, pepper and a pinch of sugar as needed.

Feel free to adjust the oil or any of the other ingredients to taste.

Serve with raw vegetables or kale chips.

Tomato Panini

This is a takeoff of the standard Panini but instead of bread, we are using tomato slices. You can certainly use gluten free bread, but what's the fun in that?

1 large Tomato, sliced crossways

Basil Pesto

Fresh Mozzarella

Preheat oven to 350 degrees F.

Arrange tomato slices on a cookie sheet. Spread a little basil pesto on each tomato slice, getting a pretty good covering.

Top with fresh mozzarella.

Place in oven and bake for 10 – 15 minutes, until mozzarella is bubble and browned.

Apple Oat Muffins

A little sweet, a little cinnamony, a whole lot of good! These are actually pretty good for you too! Have one as a snack, a dessert or even for breakfast. But you will probably want to make a double batch cause these babies go fast!

1 C Gluten Free Oat Bran
½ C Gluten Free Flour (see recipe in "Substitutions")
2 T Light Brown Sugar
2 t Gluten Free Baking Powder
1 t Cinnamon
¼ t salt
2 T Honey (clover or wildflower are best)
½ C Milk
2 T Vanilla Yogurt
1 Egg
3 T Grape Seed Oil
½ C Apple, chopped and cooked with 1 t brown sugar and ½ t cinnamon
Preheat oven to 425 degrees F. Grease your muffin tin or line it with paper liners.

In a large bowl, combine all dry ingredients. Make a well in the center of the dry ingredients and add the honey, milk, yogurt, egg and oil. Stir just until ingredients are blended.

In a small saucepan, cook apple in a little water with 1 t brown sugar and ½ t cinnamon. When apples are soft, add to the muffin mixture.

Spoon into muffin cups and bake at 425 degrees for 15 – 18 minutes. Muffins are done when a toothpick inserted in the center comes out clean.

Let Cool on a wire rack.

Variations:

Use almond or coconut milk instead of regular milk.

Add blueberries instead of apples.

Banana Nut Loaf

Ah! Warm banana nut loaf on a cool morning just does a body good. Of course, this banana nut loaf is great any time of the year. Very nice to bring to get togethers too.

1/3 C Grape Seed Oil
2/3 C Dark Brown Sugar, packed
2 Eggs
1 t Vanilla
2 T Sour Cream
1 ¾ C Gluten Free Flour (see recipe in "Substitutions")
2 t Gluten Free Baking Powder
2 t Cinnamon
1 t Guar Gum or Xanthan Gum
¼ t salt
2 Ripe Bananas, mashed
1 C Pecans or Walnuts, chopped
Preheat oven to 350 degrees F and grease a 9 X 5 inch loaf pan.

In a large bowl, cream together oil, sugar, eggs, vanilla and sour cream.

In a small bowl, mix in flour, guar gum, salt, baking powder and cinnamon.

In another small bowl, mash the bananas.

Add the dry ingredients and the banana to the wet mixture a little at a time. Alternate between the dry ingredients and the banana. When all ingredients are combined, mix thoroughly until smooth.

Gently fold in the nuts.

Spoon batter into the loaf pans and bake at 350 degrees for 45 minutes to an hour. Loaf should be golden brown and a toothpick inserted in the center will come out clean.

Spicy Seafood Cakes

These surprising little seafood cakes taste like crab cakes! Try one and you will be reaching for another! The cool thing is, they are easy to make and they are easy on the wallet!

½ - 1 pound Shrimp, chopped
1 pound Ground Chicken
1 Small Sweet Onion, chopped
2 t Garlic, minced
¾ C Brown Rice, cooked
1 can Rotel™ Tomatoes
1 C Zucchini, peeled and chopped
1 Egg, beaten with a splash of milk or cream
1 C Gluten Free Chicken Stock
Fresh Mozzarella Cheese, shredded
Paprika
Basil
Garlic Powder
Salt
Coarse Ground Black Pepper
Preheat oven to 400 degrees F. Spray a deep cookie sheet or baking pan.

Heat a little butter in a medium pan over medium high heat. Generously season the shrimp with paprika, basil garlic powder, salt and pepper. Cook until shrimp is done. Set aside.

In a medium bowl, combine the chicken, shrimp, onion, garlic, rice, Rotel and zucchini. No need to season, the seasoned shrimp, Rotel and chicken stock will provide all the flavor. Mix well.

Form "cakes" with the meat mixture and place them in the pan. They should be touching each other.

Combine the egg and about a teaspoon of cream. Whisk until well blended. Add chicken stock to make about ¾ cup. Whisk to blend.

Pour over the seafood cakes so that each one is covered.

Sprinkle cheese over each cake.

Put in the oven and bake at 400 degrees for 45 minutes to an hour. You want the ground chicken to be done.

Variations:

Use crab, lobster or fish instead of the shrimp.

Use quinoa instead of the brown rice.

Use regular crushed tomatoes with about 1 t sugar instead of the Rotel tomatoes.

Quick Snacks

When you are on the go and need some quick nourishment, try one of these snack ideas. They are fast, simple and will keep you going.

Baked Sweet Potato – Top with butter and brown sugar which is also a nice lunch or even breakfast.

Apple – Apples are high in fiber and make a great snack. There are many different types so there is certainly one that is right for you. Gala apples are super sweet while ambrosia apples are milder. Honeycrisp is nice too.

Edamame – These steamed little beans have a nutty taste. Pop them out of the shell and eat them! Delicious!

Natural Peanut Butter on Apples or Celery – You get the crunch of the apple or celery and the protein punch of peanut butter. It makes for a satisfying snack.

Toasted Seeds – Sunflower, pumpkin or other seeds get a whole new layer of flavor when you toast them. They are nice to carry with you for a quick snack on the go.

Dried Fruit – If you have a food dehydrator you can make dried fruit yourself. Otherwise, you can pick it up at the store. There are so many to choose from, apples, cherries, cranberries, blueberries, mango, apricot, the list goes on and on.

Sorbet – A nice fruit sorbet is very refreshing. Try different favors to see which you prefer.

Hard Boiled Egg – Eggs are packed with protein and other nutrients plus they provide a filling snack.

Avocado – Drizzle a little Italian dressing or salt and enjoy. Avocados have a very nice taste and texture.

Cucumber – Slice a cucumber and sprinkle with some salt or dip in a little sour cream for a refreshing summer snack.

Nuts – Walnuts, pecans, pistachios and cashews not only provide protein and are filling, they also have antidepressant qualities. Just a handful a day can help boost your mood.

Final Words

When many people are diagnosed with celiac disease or are told by their doctor that they must go gluten free, they view it as a sort of death sentence. They begin to focus on what they can't do or what they can't have. In all actuality, there is very little now that you must deprive yourself of when you go gluten free. There are some great food manufacturers out there who are committed to bringing their customers the best, most delicious gluten free food that they can.

Take some time and check them out. And check out these recipes. The recipes here should give you a good start as you begin your gluten free journey. But please, don't just take them as they are written. Experiment and explore. If you have certain spices that you like, try incorporating them into some of the recipes. If you like certain meats, try adding them or substituting them in some of the dishes. Try fish, shrimp, chicken or beef in different ways.

You will never know until you try and who knows, your family's all-time favorite dish may just hanging out, waiting to be born, right in your very kitchen. Gluten free isn't a punishment, it is just a new way of experiencing the world.

So enjoy all of the flavors and textures and new food experiences. Try some things you have never tried before. Look to your own preferences and experiences to create a dish that is truly a masterpiece. Enjoy your new food adventure as you explore new pathways to nutrition and wellness.

However, before you embark on any diet or lifestyle change, make sure you clear it with your doctor first. It is a good idea to run the program by your doctor, show him or her some sample recipes and discuss ways you can take control of your health and wellbeing. Exercise, eat right, get plenty of rest and drink lots of water. It isn't a diet, it is a lifestyle.

It is all about commitment. Make the decision, the commitment, to change your life. Whether you are going gluten free due to a health condition or because you want to lose weight or simply because you want to go more natural, make the commitment to better health.

Learn how to shop – fresh is best. Steer clear of the processed foods, or as much as you can. Avoid canned foods and stick to the foods that have the most nutritional value. Fresh vegetables, lean meats, cheeses – there's so much out there. All you have to do is reach out and grab it.

Section 2: Gluten Free Weight Loss

What is a Gluten Free Diet? Actually, it makes more sense to answer this question by first addressing what gluten is and why you may want to cut it out of your diet, especially if you're trying to lose weight. Gluten is a protein which is found in most, but not all grains, including wheat, rye, spelt (although to a lesser extent than wheat) and barley.

Gluten derived from grains is also commonly found as an ingredient, additive or binder in a variety of foods, including imitation meat products, condiments, ice cream and other products. For this reason, it's important to check food labels carefully if you're sensitive to gluten or are trying to lose weight through a gluten free diet.

A gluten free diet, as you've probably guessed by now, is a diet which is free of this protein. Although this kind of diet is restrictive in some ways, it definitely doesn't have to be something that makes you feel constantly deprived. As you'll soon find out as you read through and cook the recipes in this book, there are a lot of ways to enjoy the same dishes that you do now while leaving the gluten out.

Gluten Free Diets and Weight Loss Tips

If you've decided to adopt a gluten free diet as part of a larger weight loss program, keep in mind that all of the same rules apply as if you were following any other kind of diet. Regular exercise is an important component of any weight loss regimen and that is no different whether you're cutting gluten out of your life or not.

Additionally, you'll still have to choose what you eat carefully. There are plenty of unhealthy dietary choices out there which are gluten free and it's a mistake to eat just anything because it happens to be gluten free.

This brings us to a statistic which may surprise you. As you may know, many people choose a gluten free diet not necessarily to lose weight, but because they have celiac disease, an intolerance to gluten. According to studies, over 80% of people with gluten sensitivities who switched to a gluten free diet actually gained weight.

Why is this? Because these people didn't follow one of the most basic rules of weight loss – avoiding heavily processed foods. There's a widespread (but false) perception that if a product is labeled as gluten free, it's good for you, but that's not the case. There are many gluten free products on the market which contain nearly twice as many calories as their gluten-containing equivalents.

If you want to lose weight on a gluten free diet, it has to be a healthy diet as well as being free of gluten. This means a diet based on fresh vegetables and fruits, beans, brown rice and other healthy sources of carbohydrates as well as lean proteins. Avoid processed foods where possible and you'll probably find that you don't have a very difficult time losing weight at all.

As long as you follow these basic, common sense weight loss tips, losing weight through eating a healthy gluten free diet and getting regular exercise can be incredibly easy. Since many of the unhealthiest, most heavily processed foods in the typical western diet also contain gluten, cutting out gluten will also mean that you'll be avoiding these dietary pitfalls. Just make sure to replace these unhealthy foods with healthier choices which are also gluten free and you'll be well on your way to weight loss, more energy and better health. Without further delay, let's move on to the recipes.

Entrees

Turkey Tacos

Number of servings: 10 tacos

Ingredients:

10 corn tortillas
1 ½ lbs. lean (but not 99% fat free) ground turkey
1 medium sized onion, diced small
3 cloves of garlic, minced
½ cup low sodium chicken broth
½ cup tomato sauce (or mild salsa, if you prefer)
1 tbsp chili powder
1 tsp red wine vinegar
1 tsp oregano
1 tsp vegetable oil

Preparation:

Heat the vegetable oil in a large skillet over medium-high heat. Add the diced onion and cook for about 5 minutes or until mostly softened, stirring regularly. Add the garlic and spices and cook for another minute, stirring occasionally until the garlic becomes fragrant.

Add the ground turkey and cook for about 5 minutes, stirring constantly to break up the meat as it cooks. Cook until cooked through but still just a little bit pink. Add the tomato sauce or salsa, chicken broth, vinegar and bring to a simmer. Cook until thickened and serve hot on warmed corn tortillas with salsa, lime wedges and the condiments, toppings and garnishes of your choice.

Turkey Burgers

Number of servings: 6

Ingredients:

1lb lean ground turkey
1 small red bell pepper, diced small
1 medium sized carrot, diced small
½ of a red onion, diced small
1 small broccoli crown, minced

Preparation:

Add all of the ingredients to a large bowl and mix well to combine. Form into 6 patties and grill until they reach your desired level of doneness. Serve hot on their own or on gluten free buns with the toppings and condiments of your choice.

Thai-Style Peanut Chicken with Gluten Free Noodles

Number of servings: 4

Ingredients:

1 lb. cooked chicken breast, cut into bite sized pieces
8 ounces of rice noodles
2 cups snow peas
½ cup spicy Thai style peanut sauce (your choice)
cooking spray

Preparation:

Cook the rice noodles according to the directions on the package and set aside. Cook the snow peas in a skillet lightly coated in cooking spray over medium high heat for about 3 minutes or until cooked through and lightly seared. Add the chicken breast pieces, cooked rice noodles and peanut sauce. Reduce the heat to medium and cook until heated through, stirring regularly to combine the ingredients. Serve hot.

Fish Tacos

Number of servings: 8

Ingredients:

1 lb. halibut or tilapia filets, cut into ½" strips
8 corn tortillas
2 cups of coleslaw mix (or shredded cabbage with a little shredded carrot mixed in)
¾ cup mayonnaise
½ packed cup of cilantro, minced
1 jalapeno pepper, minced (remove the seeds for less heat)
2 tbsp rice vinegar or apple cider vinegar
3 tbsp olive oil
3 tsp cumin
3 tsp chili powder, or more to taste
juice of 1 lime
salt and black pepper, to taste
Pico de gallo and lime wedges, for serving

Preparation:

Start by preheating your oven to 325 F. Brush the tortillas with 1 tbsp of the olive oil. Wrap the oiled tortillas in aluminum foil and place in the oven to warm while you prepare the rest of the ingredients.

Add the chopped cilantro, coleslaw mix, minced jalapeno and vinegar to a bowl and mix to combine. Season to taste with salt and black pepper and set aside.

Mix together the mayonnaise, lime juice and the remaining 1 tsp of chili powder and cumin and set aside.

Remove the tortillas from the oven and divide the fish among them. Top each taco with the coleslaw mixture and a drizzle of the spiced mayonnaise. Serve hot with pico de gallo and lime wedges.

Cauliflower Crust Pizza, Hawaiian Style

Number of servings: 3 – 4 (1 12" pizza)

Ingredients:

The crust:
½ of a large cauliflower, shredded (a little more than 2 cups)
1 cup low fat mozzarella cheese, shredded
1 large egg
1 clove of garlic, minced
1 tsp oregano
a dash each of salt and black pepper
The toppings:
½ cup pizza sauce (homemade or premade)
½ cup low fat mozzarella cheese, shredded
3 thick slices of Canadian bacon, sliced into thin strips
½ cup of pineapple chunks (cut into smaller pieces, if desired)

Preparation:

Microwave the shredded cauliflower for 8 minutes in a microwave safe bowl or steam over medium-high heat in a little bit of water until softened; the microwave method is preferable, however. Allow to cool to room temperature.

Preheat your oven to 450 F and spray a pizza pan with cooking spray (or use a non-stick pan). Mix together the cauliflower and the rest of the ingredients for the crust in a bowl. Press the crust mixture into your prepared pizza pan to form a crust and lightly spray with cooking spray. Once the oven is hot, bake the crust for 15 – 17 minutes, or until it turns golden brown. Remove from the oven and increase the heat to broil.

Now you can add the toppings to your crust. Spread the sauce onto the crust, leaving a small border around the edge. Top with half of the shredded mozzarella, Canadian bacon and pineapple pieces, followed by the remainder of the cheese. Broil for 3 – 4 minutes or until the cheese melts, bubbles and browns slightly. Remove from the oven, slice and serve hot.

Sweet Potato and Black Bean Tamales

Number of servings: varies (this recipe will make approximately 20 – 24 tamales)

Ingredients:

50 dried corn husks, soaked overnight plus 3 or 4 extra
1 large poblano pepper, broiled, peeled, seeded and diced small
1 red bell pepper, diced small
1 green bell pepper, diced small
1 sweet potato, diced (may be peeled if desired)
1 can of black beans (15 – 16 ounces), drained and rinsed
1 cup diced tomatoes
½ cup cilantro, chopped
3 green onions, sliced thin
2 cloves of garlic, minced
2 tbsp olive oil
2 tsp cumin
1 tsp oregano

The dough:

2 cups masa dough
4 cups low sodium vegetable broth

2 tsp cumin
2 tsp chili powder
4 tbsp olive oil
1 tsp salt

Preparation:

Take 4 - 5 of the larger corn husks and tear them into ¼"
strips. Place the strips into a bowl of water and set aside.
Preheat your oven to 425 F. Mix together the diced
poblano, sweet potatoes, bell peppers and green onions
in a bowl. Add 1 tbsp olive oil and toss to coat. When the
oven is hot, roast the sweet potato and pepper mixture
on a foil-lined pan for about 25 minutes.

Heat 1 tbsp olive oil in a large heavy skillet over medium
heat. Saute the garlic until browned, then add the
tomatoes, roasted vegetables, black beans, cumin and
cilantro. Remove from heat and set aside while you
prepare the masa dough.

Add the masa flour, olive oil, salt, cumin and chili
powder to a food processor and blend on medium speed
to combine. Reduce the speed to low and add the broth
a little bit at a time until the mixture forms a slightly firm
dough.

Now you're ready to assemble your tamales. Lay two husks on a cutting board or other flat work surface. Place a little dough (slightly less than ¼ of a cup) at the top of two corn husks and flatten it out to cover about 2/3 of the husk, using a plastic bag to prevent the dough from sticking to your fingers. Add about 1 tbsp of the black bean mixture in the center and roll up snugly, then tie closed with one of the soaked corn husk strips. Repeat the procedure until you've used up all of the filling.

Place the tamales in a steamer, standing up with about 2 inches of water. Steam for 1 hour or until the dough easily pulls away from the husk. Serve hot with the salsa of your choice.

Steamed Shrimp and Vegetables

Number of servings: 4

Ingredients:

¾ lb. medium sized shrimp, peeled, cleaned and deveined
1 large head of bok choy, sliced about ¼" thin
1 cup snow peas
½ cup shredded carrots
1 clove of garlic, minced
a ½" piece of ginger, peeled and minced or crushed
2 tbsp reduced sodium gluten free soy sauce
1 tbsp toasted sesame oil
1 tsp rice vinegar
1 tsp chili oil
½ tsp brown sugar

Preparation:

Add the garlic, ginger, sesame and chili oil, vinegar, sugar and sesame oil to a small bowl and stir to combine. Place the shrimp in another bowl, add about 1/3 of the liquid and toss to coat. Set aside.

Steam the vegetables and shrimp until the shrimp is just

cooked through, about 10 minutes. Remove from heat, toss with the rest of the sauce and serve hot over steamed brown rice and chili paste on the side.

Gluten Free Lasagna

Number of servings: 6 - 8

Ingredients:

2 (10 ounce) boxes gluten free lasagna noodles
2 lbs. lean ground beef
3 ½ cups marinara sauce (store bought or homemade)
2 cups ricotta cheese
2 cups low fat mozzarella cheese, shredded
½ cup grated Parmesan or Romano cheese
½ cup fresh basil, finely chopped
½ cup Italian parsley, finely chopped
1 large red onion, diced small
4 cloves of garlic, minced (or more to taste)
2 eggs, lightly beaten
4 tbsp olive oil
2 tbsp Italian seasoning
1 tbsp fennel seeds, coarsely ground
2 tsp salt

Preparation:

Preheat your oven to 350 F while you get everything
ready. Bring a large stockpot 2/3 filled with cold water to
a rolling boil. Add 1 tbsp olive oil and 1 tsp salt, add 14

of the noodles and boil until al dente, about 12 – 13 minutes. Drain the noodles and rinse with cold water. Toss with 1 tbsp olive oil to prevent from sticking together and set aside.

In a large skillet, sauté the garlic and onion in 3 tbsp olive oil for 2 minutes, stirring occasionally. Add the ground beef and 1 tsp salt and cook until browned, stirring occasionally. Add the marinara sauce, half of the Italian seasoning and the fennel seeds. Stir and cook for 10 minutes, stirring as needed to keep the mixture from burning. Remove from heat and set aside.

Mix together the ricotta and Parmesan or Romano, the eggs, basil, parsley, oregano and black pepper to taste in a medium sized bowl and set aside. Now you're ready to put it all together. Spread the bottom of a 9" baking dish with the meat sauce, then a layer of lasagna noodles (it should take 4 noodles, overlapped to do this).

Follow this with a layer of the cheese mixture and a sprinkling of mozzarella. Repeat until you've used up all of the noodles, then top with the remaining sauce, mozzarella and the other 1 tbsp of Italian seasoning. Bake for about 1 hour, or until the top is golden brown. Remove from heat and allow the lasagna to rest for at least ten minutes, then slice and serve.

Butternut Squash Risotto

Number of servings: 4 – 6

Ingredients:

1 small butternut squash, peeled, seeded and diced
1 cup Arborio rice
4 cups vegetable broth, warmed
¼ cup dry sherry (not cooking sherry)
2 shallots, minced
2 cloves of garlic, minced
2 tbsp unsalted butter
2 tbsp olive oil
salt, black pepper and chopped fresh sage, to taste

Preparation:

Heat the olive oil and butter in a large saucepan over medium heat. Once the oil and butter are hot, add the shallots and a little black pepper and sauté until softened, about 3 minutes. Add the garlic and a pinch of salt, stir and cook for another minute. Add the cubed squash and cook for about 10 minutes or until the squash starts to soften, about 10 minutes. Add the rice and cook for another 1 – 2 minutes, stirring regularly to prevent burning.

Add the sherry and cook until the alcohol cooks off and the rice absorbs the remaining liquid. Add ½ cup of vegetable broth and continue to cook at a simmer, stirring constantly until the broth is absorbed. Repeat until the broth is all absorbed and the rice is tender and takes on a creamy texture, 15 – 20 minutes. Sprinkle with chopped sage and serve hot.

Seared Ahi Tuna with Grilled Vegetable Quinoa Salad

Number of servings: 8

Ingredients:

2 lbs. ahi tuna
2 cups dry quinoa
2 zucchini, sliced lengthwise
2 yellow summer squash, sliced lengthwise
2 small eggplants, sliced lengthwise
2 large Portabella mushrooms, sliced
1 large yellow or white onion, sliced
4 Roma tomatoes, diced
4 ½ cups low sodium vegetable stock
4 tbsp olive oil
2 tbsp rice vinegar or apple cider vinegar
2 tsp dried chives (or 2 tbsp fresh chives, if available)
2 tsp tarragon
2 tsp thyme
salt and black pepper, to taste
1 head of raddichio, for serving
cooking spray

Preparation:

Rinse the quinoa well in a strainer while you bring the vegetable stock to a boil in a medium saucepan. Add the quinoa and thyme, reduce heat, cover and simmer until the quinoa absorbs the liquid and becomes fluffy, about 15 minutes. Fluff the quinoa with a fork and set aside.

Spray a skillet with cooking spray and cook the vegetables over medium heat until they're tender. Remove from heat and set aside. After giving the vegetables a few minutes to cool, dice them into small pieces. Add the diced vegetables, quinoa, tomatoes and remaining herbs to a bowl and toss to mix. Add black pepper to taste, stir again and set aside.

Season the tuna with black pepper and brush with 1 tbsp olive oil while you heat a nonstick skillet over high heat. Sear the tuna on each side and remove from heat. Transfer the tuna to a cutting board and cut into thin slices with a sharp knife. Arrange radicchio leaves on serving plates, topped with quinoa salad and a portion of the tuna slices. Serve immediately.

Blackened Shrimp Nachos

Number of servings: 4

Ingredients:

½ lb. cooked shrimp, tails removed
½ of a red bell pepper, diced small
½ cup shredded Monterey Jack or cheddar cheese
1 small jalapeno, sliced thinly
2 tbsp chopped cilantro
2 tbsp Italian dressing
gluten-free tortilla chips
1 tsp sweet (Hungarian) paprika
2 tsp salt
1 tsp black pepper
1 tsp garlic powder
½ tsp cayenne pepper, or more to taste
salsa, for serving

Preparation:

Preheat your oven to 375 F. Heat a large, non-stick
skillet over high heat until very hot. Add ½ of the Italian
dressing, the diced bell peppers and the spices. Cook for
about 1 – 1 ½ minutes or until the pepper begins to look
roasted, stirring regularly. Add the shrimp and cook,

stirring regularly until the shrimp is well coated with the spice mixture and cooked through. Add the remaining dressing, remove from heat and set aside.

Arrange tortilla chips in a single layer on a baking sheet, topped with half of the shrimp and cheese. Add a second layer of tortilla chips, then the remaining shrimp and cheese, then top with the sliced jalapenos. Bake for about 10 minutes, or until the cheese is melted and slightly browned. Remove from heat and top with chopped cilantro. Serve at once with the salsa of your choice.

Gluten-Free Beef Stew

Number of servings: 6 - 8

Ingredients:

1 lb. lean beef stew meat
1 lb. red potatoes, cubed
2 cups diced tomatoes
2 cups beef stock
1 cup fresh or frozen peas
1 cup fresh or frozen corn
1 medium sized yellow onion, diced
3 medium sized carrots, sliced
3 cloves of garlic, sliced
2 tbsp brandy (optional)
2 tbsp rice flour
2 tbsp potato starch
1 tbsp olive oil
1 tsp each thyme and oregano
salt and black pepper, to taste

Preparation:

Mix together the rice flour, potato starch, salt, pepper
and herbs in a large bowl with a lid. Add the beef, close
and shake well to coat. Heat the olive oil in a large skillet

over medium high heat. Place the beef in the skillet (save the remaining flour mixture for later) and cook for about 3 minutes per side or until just browned. Add the brandy (if using) and cook for another minute. Remove from heat and set aside.

Add the beef stock, onions, carrots and tomatoes to a large saucepan or stock pot over medium heat. Add 1 tbsp of the remaining flour mixture and stir to coat. Add the beef, reduce to a simmer and cook, covered for 2 hours. Add the potatoes and cook for another 30 – 35 minutes or until the potatoes are tender. Add the corn and peas and cook for 10 – 15 minutes or until heated through. Season to taste with salt and black pepper and serve hot.

Orange Chicken

Number of servings: 4

Ingredients:

2 skinless, boneless chicken breasts, cut into bite sized pieces
2 cups cooked brown rice, kept warm
3 cups shredded Savoy cabbage or green cabbage

1 red bell pepper, sliced into strips
1 cup small broccoli florets
4 green onions, trimmed and sliced thinly
1 cup San-J brand orange sauce
¼ cup corn starch
2 tbsp canola oil
chili sauce, to taste

Preparation:

Toss the chicken and corn starch in a bowl or bag to coat while you heat the oil in a large skillet or wok over medium heat. Add the chicken pieces and cook, stirring occasionally until the chicken is cooked through and slightly crisp on the outside; this will take 5 minutes or less. Remove the chicken and set aside.

Add the vegetables to the skillet and cook for about 5 minutes or until slightly reduced and heated through, stirring regularly. Return the chicken to the pan along with the orange sauce and a little chili sauce. Stir and continue cooking for another 1 - 2 minutes or until heated through. Serve hot over brown rice.

Tuna Casserole

Number of servings: 4

Ingredients:

8 ounces gluten free pasta (your choice, but small shells work the best)
1 12 ounce can of tuna in water, drained and broken up into small pieces
1 small yellow onion, diced
½ of a red bell pepper, diced small
1 cup frozen or fresh peas
1 cup shredded sharp cheddar cheese
1 cup gluten free bread or cracker crumbs
1 cup gluten free cream of mushroom soup
1 ½ cups milk
4 tbsp rice flour
2 tbsp butter
1 tbsp olive oil
salt and black pepper, to taste

Preparation:

Preheat your oven to 350 F. Cook the pasta according to the directions on the package. Just before the pasta is done, add the peas. Drain and rinse in cold water, then pour into a large bowl and set aside.

Melt the butter in a saucepan over medium heat, then add the onion and bell pepper and sauté for about 3 minutes, stirring occasionally. Add the rice flour, stir to combine and continue to cook for another 3 minutes, stirring regularly. Add the mushroom soup, milk and salt and pepper to taste. Whisk to combine. Reduce to a simmer and continue stirring until the mixture thickens.

Pour the thickened sauce over the pasta and peas, followed by the tuna and half of the cheese. Stir to combine. Pour the mixture into a 9" x 13" baking dish and top with the other half of the cheese. Mix together the bread or cracker crumbs and olive oil until combined and sprinkle over the casserole. Bake for 40 minutes or until the casserole is bubbling and nicely browned. Remove from the oven and allow to rest for 5 minutes before serving.

Goat Cheese Ravioli

Number of servings: 4

Ingredients:

8 gluten free lasagna sheets
1 large (28 ounce) can of whole tomatoes with juice
2 tbsp unsalted butter
2 tbsp minced shallots
1 tbsp olive oil
1 tsp Italian seasoning
salt, black pepper and red pepper flakes, to taste
The filling:
1 cup goat cheese
¼ cup arugula leaves, chopped
1 clove of garlic, minced or crushed
2 tbsp olive oil
1 tsp lemon zest
1 tsp black pepper
salt and black pepper, to taste

Preparation:

Cook the pasta according to the directions on the
package, drain and rinse in cold water. Transfer the
cooked pasta to a cutting board and slice each noodle

into 3 pieces. Place between damp towels and set aside.

Next, make your sauce. Heat 1 tbsp of olive oil in a medium sized saucepan over medium heat. Saute the shallots, red pepper flakes (if desired) and Italian seasoning until the shallots turn transparent, stirring occasionally. Add the tomatoes, reduce the heat to low and simmer for 30 minutes, stirring regularly until the tomatoes break down and form a sauce. Add the butter and continue simmering until it melts, stirring to combine. Season to taste with salt and black pepper, remove from heat and cover to keep warm.

Preheat your oven to 375 F and start making the filling. Saute the garlic in the other tbsp of olive oil over medium heat until golden brown, 2 – 3 minutes. Add the arugula, lemon zest and black pepper and cook for about 2 minutes or until the arugula is wilted, stirring frequently. Transfer the arugula to a cutting board, allow to cool for a few minutes, chop finely and transfer to a bowl along with the goat cheese. Stir to combine and set aside.

Spray a 9" x 13" baking dish with cooking spray and place half of the pasta squares in the dish. Top each square with about 1 tbs of the filling and cover with another pasta square. Pour the sauce over the ravioli and bake for about 15 minutes, or until heated through. Remove from the oven and serve at once.

Shrimp and Tofu Pad Thai

Number of servings: 4

Ingredients:

½ lb. medium sized shrimp, cleaned, peeled and deveined (if frozen, thaw first)
8 oz. rice noodles
8 oz. firm tofu, cubed
3 tbsp vegetable oil
2 eggs, lightly beaten
1 small onion, thinly sliced
2 cloves of garlic, minced
1 cup shredded carrots
1 cup gluten free Pad Thai sauce (your choice)
2 tbsp chopped cilantro, 2 tbsp chopped roasted peanuts, green onion slices and lime wedges, for garnish

Preparation:

Cook the rice noodles as per the directions on the package. Rinse with cold water in a colander and set aside. Heat 1 tbsp of the vegetable oil in a large skillet or wok over high heat. Add the eggs and scramble, stirring constantly to prevent burning. Remove from the skillet or wok, place in a bowl and set aside.

Add the rest of the vegetable oil to the skillet or wok and heat. Add the shrimp and onion and cook, stirring frequently, until the shrimp are cooked through and opaque. Add the garlic and ginger and cook for another minute, then transfer to the bowl along with the eggs and reduce the heat to low. Return the noodles to the skillet or wok along with the Pad Thai sauce and stir to combine. Return the shrimp, eggs, followed by the rest of the ingredients. Serve immediately, garnished with the peanuts, cilantro, green onions and lime wedges.

Tuna Melt Tostadas

Number of servings: 2

Ingredients:

1/3 cup tuna in water, drained
2 corn tortillas
1 tsp mayonnaise
1 tsp pickle relish or diced dill pickle
½ tsp brown mustard
4 tbsp shredded cheddar cheese
cooking spray

Preparation:

Start by preheating your oven to 400 F. Mix together the tuna, mustard, mayonnaise and relish or diced pickle in a bowl. Set aside. Lightly coat a baking sheet with cooking spray and place the tortillas on the prepared baking sheet. Lightly spray the tops of the tortillas and bake until they begin to brown and become crisp. Remove from the oven, top with the tuna mixture and shredded cheddar cheese. Return to the oven and bake until the cheese is melted to your liking. Remove from the oven and serve immediately.

Mussels over Pasta

Number of servings: 4

Ingredients:

2 lbs. live mussels, scrubbed well and rinsed
8 ounces gluten free linguini or fettucine, cooked
1 small celery stalk, diced
½ of a small white or yellow onion, diced
2 cloves of garlic, minced
juice of ½ lemon
1 cup water
2 tbsp Italian parsley, chopped
2 tbsp fresh basil, chopped
2 tbsp olive oil (use extra virgin olive oil for this recipe, if
you have it on hand)
salt and black pepper, to taste

Preparation:

First, make sure that your mussels are still alive. Tap
them lightly against the side of your sink; they should
make a dull sound, not a hollow sound – they'll also
close their shells if they're alive. Scrub the mussels well,
taking care to remove their bears and rinse well. Set
aside.

In a large saucepan, sauté the garlic and onion in olive oil over medium heat until the garlic turns golden brown. Add the celery, parsley, water, lemon juice and a little salt and pepper and bring the mixture to a boil. Add the basil and mussels, cover and steam for 5 – 10 minutes, or until all of the mussels have opened. Remove from heat and discard any unopened mussels. Serve in bowls over a portion of the cooked pasta.

Pork Chops With Mushroom – Pomegranate Sauce

Number of servings: 4

Ingredients:

1 lb. pork (or lamb) chops rubbed with 1 tsp thyme
1 cup button or crimini mushrooms, sliced
½ of a medium-sized yellow onion, minced
3 cloves of garlic, minced
2 tbsp olive oil
salt and black pepper, to taste

The sauce:

1 cup of pomegranate juice
1 tbsp rice vinegar
1 tbsp corn starch
½ tablespoon honey

Preparation:

Preheat your oven to 350 F. Heat the olive oil a large, heavy skillet (a cast iron skillet works well) over medium-high heat and sauté the mushrooms, onions and garlic until tender. Transfer to a bowl and set aside. Add the pork chops to the skillet and cook for 6 minutes per side, then remove from the pan. Whisk together the ingredients for the pomegranate sauce and pour into the pan. Deglaze the pan briefly and return the pork to the skillet.

Return the mushroom mixture to the skillet and transfer to the oven to cook for another 10 – 15 minutes, or until the pork chops are cooked through and the sauce is thickened. Remove from the oven and serve hot over brown rice or gluten free pasta.

Stuffed Potatoes

Number of servings: 2

Ingredients:

2 large russet potatoes, washed and pierced with a fork
2 hardboiled eggs, mashed
4 tbsp shredded Manchego cheese
2 tbsp diced tomato
black pepper, to taste
The tuna salad:
1/2 cup tuna in water, drained
2 tbsp mayonnaise
1 tbsp diced celery
1 tbsp green onion slices
1 tsp Dijon mustard
salt and black pepper, to taste

Preparation:

Bake or microwave the potatoes. While they're cooking, combine the ingredients for the tuna salad and refrigerate until you're ready to use it. Slice the potatoes lengthwise and use a fork to mash the insides. Stir in the cheese, followed by the tuna salad, then the mashed egg and finally the diced tomato. Season to taste with black pepper and serve immediately.

Tuscan Style Chicken with Mushrooms

Number of servings: 4

Ingredients:

1 whole fryer chicken (3 – 3 ½ lbs.), disjointed
2 cups cooked gluten free pasta (your choice)
¾ cup sliced crimini mushrooms
¾ cup diced carrots
¾ cup water
½ cup diced celery
¼ cup olive oil
3 tbsp chopped Italian parsley
2 cloves of garlic, chopped
1 medium sized tomato, diced
1 tbsp red wine vinegar
½ tsp basil
½ tsp salt
½ tsp black pepper, or more to taste

Preparation:

Heat the olive oil in a large skillet over medium heat; once the oil is hot, add the chicken and fry until browned on both sides. Move the chicken over to the side of the pan and add the mushrooms. Cook until the mushrooms release their water and turn slightly golden, about 3 minutes. Add the celery, garlic and carrots and cook for another 3 minutes, stirring regularly. Add the salt, pepper, basil, vinegar, tomato and parsley and cook for 3 more minutes, stirring occasionally. Add the water, reduce the heat to low and cover. Cook, covered for 25 minutes. Remove the chicken and transfer to serving plates. Add the pasta to the skillet and stir to combine with the vegetables. Cook for 1 -2 minutes or until the pasta is heated through. Serve immediately.

Stuffed Cabbage

Number of servings: 4 - 6 (2 -3 cabbage leaves per serving)

Ingredients:

1 lb. lean ground turkey
12 large green cabbage leaves
1 cup white or parboiled brown rice, uncooked
½ tsp salt
¼ black pepper, or more to taste
The sauce:
4 cups tomato sauce (your choice or homemade)
4 cups of reserved water from cooking the cabbage
½ tsp cinnamon
½ tsp salt

Preparation:

Core a head of cabbage and soak in a large bowl (or clean sink) full of hot water for 10 minutes. Remove and carefully peel off 12 cabbage leaves or a few extra in case you end up tearing one while stuffing them. Bring 6 cups of water to a boil in a large pot and add the cabbage leaves. Cook for a few minutes to blanch and soften, but not thoroughly cook the leaves. Remove and transfer to a plate. Reserve 4 cups of the cooking water and discard the rest.

Mix together the ground turkey in a bowl with the rice, salt and pepper. Add about ¼ cup of the turkey mixture to the inside of each leaf and roll up, burrito style, to close. Repeat the process until you've used up all of the filling.

Add the tomato sauce to the pot with the reserved cooking water and lay your extra cabbage leaves on the bottom to prevent the rolls from sticking to the pot. Arrange the cabbage rolls in the pot, bring to a boil and then reduce the heat to a low simmer and cook for 35 – 40 minutes. Remove the rolls carefully and serve hot.

Brazil Nut-Crusted Tilapia

Number of servings: 3

Ingredients:

3 tilapia filets (4 – 6 ounces each)
1 cup brazil nuts, chopped
3 tbsp crushed gluten free corn flakes
3 tbsp olive oil
3 tbsp milk
salt and black pepper, to taste

Preparation:

Start by preheating your oven to 350 F. Mix together the brazil nuts, crushed corn flakes and some salt and pepper on a large plate. Pour the milk onto another plate. Dip the filets in milk, then roll in the brazil nut mixture until thickly coated. Spread the olive oil on a baking sheet and add the filets. Bake for about 20 minutes or until the fish flakes easily with a fork. Remove from the oven and serve at once.

Appetizers, Side Dishes and Soups

Cucumber - Chickpea Bruschetta

Number of servings: varies

Ingredients:

1 large or 2 small cucumbers, sliced about ¼" – 1/3" thick
1 can of chickpeas, drained, rinsed and mashed
juice of ½ lemon
finely diced tomatoes and red onions, chopped dill and black pepper, for garnish
salt and black pepper, to taste

Preparation:

Mix the mashed chickpeas with lemon juice and a little salt and black pepper, stirring well to combine. Spread the cucumber slices with the chickpeas, transfer to a serving plate and set aside. In a bowl, mix together the tomatoes, onion, herbs and salt and black pepper to taste. Add a small spoonful of the mixture to each cucumber slice and serve immediately or refrigerate for a few hours and serve chilled.

Vinegar Slaw

Number of servings: varies

Ingredients:

2 cups shredded cabbage (green, red or Savoy, your choice)
½ cup shredded carrot
2 tbsp honey
2 tbsp apple cider vinegar, or more to taste
2 tbsp water
salt and black pepper, to taste

Preparation:

Nothing could be easier than preparing this recipe. Simply add all of the ingredients to a large bowl, stir or toss well to combine. Serve at once or refrigerate for a few hours or overnight to allow the flavors to blend.

Balsamic Glazed Roasted Vegetables

Number of servings: 4

Ingredients:

10 large Brussels sprouts, trimmed and halved
4 large carrots, quartered and cut into 2" slices
3 cloves of garlic, minced
1 large shallot, minced
½ cup balsamic vinegar
2 tbsp butter
2 sprigs of fresh thyme or 1 tsp dried thyme

Preparation:

Preheat your oven to 400 F. Melt the butter in a small saucepan over medium – high heat. Add the garlic and shallots and sauté for about 3 minutes or until the garlic starts to become tender. Add the thyme and cook for another minute, stirring occasionally. Add the vinegar and allow the mixture to reduce for about 3 minutes. Allow the sauce to rest for a few minutes, then toss in a large bowl with the vegetables.

Line a baking sheet with foil and spread out the vegetables on the sheet. Bake for 25 minutes, remove from the oven and serve hot.

Quinoa Ranch Salad

Number of servings: 6

Ingredients:

2 cups water
1 red bell pepper, diced
1 yellow bell pepper, diced
4 green onions, trimmed and sliced thinly
1 ½ cups cooked black beans (drain and rinse if using
canned beans)
1 cup quinoa, uncooked
1 cup finely diced sweet potato
1 cup gluten free ranch dressing (your choice or
homemade)
½ cup pepitas
¼ cup Italian parsley, chopped
salt and black pepper, to taste

Preparation:

Rinse the quinoa well in a colander, place in a medium
saucepan and add the water. Bring to a boil briefly,
reduce the heat to simmer and cook, covered for about
12 minutes or until the quinoa has absorbed almost all
of the water. Remove from heat but keep covered and

allow to rest for 10 minutes before removing the lid and placing into your freezer to cool.

Place the remaining ingredients in a large bowl, add the quinoa and sweet potato once cooled and mix well. Pour the ranch dressing over the salad and stir well to coat. Serve at once or refrigerate, covered and serve chilled.

Sunflower Seed Hummus

Number of servings: varies

Ingredients:

2 (15 ounce) cans of chickpeas, drained and rinsed well
1 cup unsalted sunflower seeds (roasted or raw, your choice)
6 cloves of garlic
1 ½ tbsp olive oil (use extra virgin olive oil for this recipe)
2 tbsp water
juice of 1 lemon or more to taste
salt and black pepper, to taste
a pinch of paprika

Preparation:

Add the garlic and sunflower seeds to a food processor and pulse until they reach the consistency of a coarse meal. Add the remaining ingredients and process until it reaches the consistency you like. Add a little extra water or lemon juice if needed. Season to taste with salt and black pepper, transfer to a serving bowl and sprinkle with paprika and sunflower seeds. Serve at once or refrigerate, covered and serve chilled.

Zucchini and Leek Soup

Number of servings: 6 - 8

Ingredients:

5 leeks, green parts removed, sliced and thoroughly cleaned
6 cups sliced zucchini or yellow summer squash
4 cups of low sodium vegetable or chicken stock
4 cloves of garlic, minced
½ cup coconut milk
½ cup dry white wine
3 tbsp olive oil
1 tbsp apple cider vinegar
1 tbsp dill
salt and black pepper, to taste

Preparation:

Heat a very large saucepan or stock pot over medium heat for 30 seconds to one minute. Add the olive oil and continue to heat for 1 minute. Add the zucchini, leeks and garlic and cook for about 5 minutes, stirring occasionally.

Add the wine and vegetable or chicken stock and bring

the soup to a boil. Reduce the heat to a simmer and cook, covered for 30 minutes. Add the vinegar, coconut milk, dill and a little salt and pepper and heat through. Transfer the soup to a blender in batches (or use a hand blender) and blend until smooth and creamy. Season to taste with salt and black pepper and serve hot.

Cranberry Glazed Carrots

Number of servings: 6

Ingredients:

2 lbs. baby carrots
½ cup cranberry sauce (whole berry or jellied, your choice)
2 tbsp butter
2 tbsp brown sugar
1 tbsp lemon juice
salt and black pepper, to taste

Preparation:

Add the carrots to a large saucepan with about 1" of water. Bring to a boil, then reduce the heat and simmer, covered for 10 minutes, or until the carrots are tender. Drain and transfer to a bowl. Add the remaining ingredients to the pan and cook over medium heat, stirring regularly, until the mixture is smooth. Return the carrots to the pan, stir well to coat and continue cooking until the carrots are heated through. Serve at once.

Grilled Radicchio with Goat Cheese

Number of servings: 8

Ingredients:

2 heads of radicchio
2 cloves of garlic, minced
½ cup olive oil (use extra virgin olive oil, if you have it on hand)
½ cup goat cheese
¼ cup balsamic vinegar
2 tbsp chopped basil
salt and black pepper, to taste

Preparation:

Quarter the radicchio (don't remove the stem end) and soak in ice water for 1 hour. Meanwhile, whisk together the garlic, vinegar and olive oil in a bowl and set aside. Start your grill, drain the radicchio and place on paper towels to soak up excess water. Open up each quarter, spoon in a portion of the dressing and season with a little salt and pepper.

Once the grill is ready, cook the radicchio for about 3 minutes per side. Remove from the grill and stuff with goat cheese and chopped basil. If there's any of the dressing left, spoon it on top before serving.

Tex-Mex Style Summer Squash

Number of servings: 4

Ingredients:

2 cups cubed yellow summer squash or zucchini
1 cup cooked brown rice, cooled to room temperature
½ cup refried black beans
1/3 cup water
1 tbsp chopped cilantro
1 tsp cumin
salt and black pepper, to taste
salsa, for serving (your choice)

Preparation:

Bring the water to a boil in a medium sized saucepan.
Add the squash and a little salt and black pepper.
Reduce to a simmer and cook for 5 minutes or until the
squash is just beginning to become tender. Add the rice,
cumin, refried beans and chopped cilantro. Cook for
another 2 – 3 minutes to heat through, stirring
occasionally. Serve hot with the salsa of your choice.

Butternut Squash Soup

Number of servings: 4 - 6

Ingredients:

1 large butternut squash (about 2 lbs.)
2 cups of low sodium chicken or vegetable stock
1 cup of diced yellow onion
½ cup thinly sliced carrots
¼ cup heavy cream
2 cloves of garlic, chopped
½ of a jalapeno pepper, minced
2 tablespoons peanut oil
1 tsp cumin
salt and black pepper, to taste

Preparation:

Halve the squash lengthwise and remove the seeds and surrounding pulp. Peel the squash and cut into 1" cubes. Heat the peanut oil in a large saucepan or stock pot over medium heat. Once the oil is hot, add the garlic and onion and cook until they start to brown, stirring frequently (about 5 minutes). Add the carrots, cumin and a little salt and pepper and cook for another minute, stirring occasionally.

Add the jalapeno, squash and chicken or vegetable stock and bring to a boil. Reduce the heat and simmer, covered, for 20 minutes or until the squash is tender. Remove from heat and puree in batches in a blender or use a hand blender to blend the soup until smooth. Return the soup to the pot over medium heat, whisk in the cream and season to taste with salt and black pepper. Remove from heat and serve hot.

Gluten-free Pot Stickers

Number of servings: 6 (about 24 pot stickers)

Ingredients:

The wrappers:
1 cup brown rice flour
2/3 cup boiling water
½ cup tapioca flour
¼ cup white rice flour
2 tbsp canola oil
½ tsp salt
¼ tsp xanthan gum
cornstarch, for rolling
The filling:
1 lb. lean ground pork
2 green onions, trimmed and sliced thinly
2 cloves of garlic, minced
1 tsp fresh ginger, minced or crushed
1 tbsp sesame oil
salt and black pepper, to taste

Preparation:

Add all of the ingredients to a large bowl and mix well to combine. Set aside. Mix together the dry ingredients for the wrappers and add boiling water a little bit at a time, mixing with a chopstick. Once the dough is cool enough to handle, knead gently with your hands until the dough reaches the consistency of modeling clay (think Play-Doh). Roll the dough into a log and cut in half. Place one half in a plastic bag until you're ready to use it.

Cut the other half of the dough into 12 pieces and roll each piece into a flat circle of dough. Sprinkle each with corn starch and roll out in between two sheets of plastic wrap until very thin. Roll out 6 wrappers at a time. Brush a wrapper with a little water and add 2 tsp of the filling to the middle, fold over and seal. Set aside. Repeat the process until you've made all 24 pot stickers.

Heat the oil in a large skillet over medium heat, add as many pot stickers as will fit and cook for 2 minutes or until slightly browned. Add ¼ cup water and cook, covered for 8 minutes. Remove the cover and cook uncovered for 3 more minutes or until well browned. Repeat until you've cooked all of the pot stickers and serve hot with the condiments of your choice.

Creamy Cauliflower Soup

Number of servings: 2

Ingredients:

1 ½ fresh or frozen cauliflower florets
1 cup of low sodium chicken or vegetable broth
3 wedges of Laughing Cow (or other brand) light cheese
with garlic and herbs
2 tbsp low fat cheddar cheese
1 tbsp chopped chives
1 tbsp cooked, crumbled turkey bacon
salt and black pepper, to taste

Preparation:

Bring the cauliflower and vegetable or chicken broth to a
boil in a medium saucepan. Reduce to a simmer and
cook, covered for about 15 minutes, or until the
cauliflower starts to fall apart (the cooking time will be
less if you're using frozen cauliflower). Remove from
heat and add to a blender with the garlic and herb
cheese and a little salt and black pepper. Blend until
smooth and transfer to a bowl. Stir in the chives and
cheddar cheese, divide among 2 bowls and top each
with half of the crumbled turkey bacon. Serve

immediately.

Prosciutto Wrapped Basil Shrimp

Number of servings: 4 (5 shrimp per serving)

Ingredients:

20 large shrimp, peeled, deveined and cleaned (and thawed, if frozen)
10 very thinly sliced pieces of prosciutto
1 tbsp of chopped basil
1 tsp olive oil (use extra virgin olive oil for this recipe if you have some on hand)
1 tsp lemon zest
½ tsp salt
½ tsp crushed red pepper flakes
a pinch of black pepper
cooking spray
lemon wedges, for serving

Preparation:

Start by preheating your oven to broil. Add the shrimp, olive oil, chopped basil, lemon zest, salt, black pepper and red pepper flakes. Toss to coat the shrimp with the other ingredients and set aside until later.

Lay out the slices of prosciutto on a large, clean work

surface and cut each slice lengthwise in half to make 20 pieces of prosciutto in total. Wrap each shrimp with a slice of prosciutto, with the tail still hanging out. Thread the shrimp on a skewer and repeat the process until you have 4 skewers, each with 5 shrimp.

Now you're ready to cook the shrimp. Lightly coat a baking sheet with cooking spray, place the skewers on the sheet and place under the broiler. Broil for two minutes per side, remove the shrimp from the oven and serve at once with lemon wedges on the side.

Breakfast

Gluten Free Spinach Quiche

Number of servings: 6

Ingredients:

1 prebaked gluten free 9" pie crust (you can find these at health food stores)
1 cup prewashed baby spinach leaves, tightly packed
2/3 cup shredded Swiss or Jarlsberg cheese
3 large eggs
1 ¼ cups heavy cream
1 tsp salt
1 tsp black pepper
½ tsp nutmeg

Preparation:

Start by preheating your oven to 375 F. Whisk together the eggs, cream, nutmeg, black pepper and salt. Sprinkle half of the cheese on the bottom of the pie crust, followed by half of the spinach leaves. Pour about 2/3 of the egg mixture over the spinach, followed by the rest of the spinach and cheese, then the remaining eggs.

Bake for 30 minutes or until the quiche is set in the middle and golden brown on top. Remove from the oven and allow to rest for 5 – 10 minutes before slicing and serving.

Gluten Free Croissants

Number of servings: 12 croissants

Ingredients:

8 large eggs
2 cups of water
1 1/3 cup brown rice flour
1 cup of cold, unsalted butter
2/3 cup potato starch
2 tbsp sugar
1 tsp salt
cooking spray

Preparation:

Preheat your oven to 450 F and lightly coat a large baking sheet with cooking spray. Add the water and butter to a large saucepan and bring to a boil until the butter is melted. Whisk to combine and remove from heat.

Mix the dry ingredients in a large bowl and then add the water and shortening mixture. Stir until the dough pulls together into a ball. Allow the dough to cool for 10 – 15 minutes. Add the eggs one at a time, beating each egg into the dough until thoroughly combined. You should now have very sticky dough.

Spoon about 1/3 cup of dough onto the baking sheet for each croissant. Bake for 20 minutes. Reduce the heat to 350 F and bake for another 10 minutes. Remove from the oven, allow them to cool to room temperature and serve with the toppings of your choice. Individually wrap leftover croissants and refrigerate.

Pumpkin Muffins with Maple – Cream Cheese Filling

Number of servings: 12

Ingredients:

2 large eggs
1 cup brown rice flour
1 cup canned pumpkin
¾ cup sugar
½ cup canola oil
1/3 cup potato flour
¼ cup almond milk
4 tbsp tapioca starch
1 ½ tsp cinnamon
¾ tsp allspice
½ tsp ground ginger
½ tsp salt
1 tsp baking soda
¾ tsp xanthan gum (use corn starch if you can't find this)
½ tsp baking powder

The filling:

½ cup low fat cream cheese, softened at room temperature

¼ cup powdered sugar

2 tbsp maple syrup

Preparation:

Start by preheating your oven to 350 F. Line cupcake or muffin tins with liners. Mix together all of the dry ingredients in a large bowl until well combined. Mix together the eggs and sugar in a separate bowl until smooth. Add the remainder of the wet ingredients and mix until smooth. Stir the dry ingredients slowly into the wet ingredients until well combined. Fill each muffin liner about ¾ full and set aside.

Now you can make the filling. Add the cream cheese, powdered sugar and maple syrup to a food processor and blend until very smooth. Spoon about 1 tbsp of the filling into each muffin liner. Bake for 25 minutes or until a toothpick inserted into the center of a muffin comes out dry or with just a few crumbs.

Remove the muffins from the oven and allow to cool in the tin for 5 – 10 minutes, then transfer the muffins to a cooling rack to cool to room temperature before serving.

Coconut Flour Pancakes

Number of servings: 6

Ingredients:

3 large eggs
3 tbsp coconut flour
3 tbsp coconut oil
3 tbsp coconut milk
1 tsp brown sugar
½ tsp baking soda
¼ tsp salt
a little canola oil, for cooking

Preparation:

In a medium sized bowl, whisk together the oil, eggs, coconut milk, salt and sugar. Mix in the remaining ingredients and add a little water until the batter reaches your desired consistency.

Heat a little canola oil in a frying pan or skillet. Pour in ¼ cup per pancake and cook until done on both sides. Serve hot with the toppings of your choice.

Turnip Hash

Number of servings: 4

Ingredients:

2 medium sized turnips, trimmed and grated
1 medium russet potato, grated
½ of a medium sized yellow or red onion, diced
1 tbsp olive oil
1 tbsp chopped Italian parsley
salt and black pepper, to taste

Preparation:

Mix together the shredded turnips and potatoes in a large bowl, then add the diced onion and a little salt and black pepper. Toss again to combine. Heat the olive oil in a large, heavy skillet over medium – high heat. Once the oil is hot, transfer the turnips and potatoes and cook for about 12 minutes, flipping over halfway through. Cook until crisp on both sides, sprinkle with chopped parsley and serve hot.

Crepes

Number of servings: 3 (2 crepes per serving)
1 large egg
2/3 cup whole milk
1/3 cup corn starch
2 tsp melted butter
a pinch of salt
a little canola oil, for cooking

Preparation:

Add all of the ingredients to a blender and mix until thoroughly combined. Drizzle a little bit of oil into a large, heavy skillet over medium high heat. Remove from heat and pour in about 2 tbsp of batter, swirling the skillet to spread the batter. Cook for about 30 seconds, or until the crepe browns around the edges and starts to pull away from the sides of the skillet. If the crepe doesn't brown, increase the heat slightly.

Lift the edge of the crepe gently with a spatula, grab with your fingers or tongs and flip over. Cook for another 20 seconds and transfer to a plate. Repeat the process until you've used up all of the batter. Enjoy with the sweet or savory fillings and toppings of your choice.

Berry Cornbread Muffins

Number of servings:

Ingredients:

1 large egg
1 cup fresh or frozen mixed berries, your choice
1 cup milk or almond milk
1 cup gluten free flour
¾ cup cornmeal
½ cup corn flour
¼ cup sugar
¼ cup canola oil
4 tsp baking powder
1 tsp vanilla extract
¼ tsp salt
zest of 1 lemon

Preparation:

Start by preheating your oven to 400 F. Line a 12 cup muffin tin with liners. Combine all of the dry ingredients in a large bowl and mix well to combine. Mix all of the wet ingredients until thoroughly combined in a separate bowl. Add the wet ingredients to the dry ingredients a little at a time, mixing until they're just combined. Fold in the berries gently. Divide the batter among the lined muffin cups, sprinkle with lemon zest and bake for 18 – 20 minutes, or until a toothpick inserted in the center of a muffin comes out clean. Allow to cool for at least five minutes, then transfer to a wire rack to cool to room temperature before serving.

Quinoa and Corn Cakes

Number of servings: 5 – 6 (10 – 12 cakes)

Ingredients:

1 cup cooked quinoa
1 large egg
2 scallions, trimmed and sliced thinly
½ cup water
½ cup vegetable broth
½ cup fresh or frozen corn (thaw first if using frozen corn)
1/3 cup diced red bell pepper
¼ cup shredded low fat mozzarella
¼ cup gluten free flour (your choice)
2 tbsp corn flour
2 tbsp milk or almond milk
½ tsp salt
½ tsp black pepper
a little canola oil, for frying
salsa, for serving (your choice)

Preparation:

Beat the egg in a medium sized bowl and then add the remaining ingredients (except for the canola oil). Mix well to combine. If the batter is too wet, add another tbsp of flour. Heat a little canola oil in a large non-stick pan. When the oil is hot, add ¼ cup of the batter and press with a spatula. Cook as many at a time as you can while still leaving room between the cakes. Cook for about 3 minutes per side, or until golden brown. Serve immediately with the salsa of your choice.

Gluten Free Banana Bread

Number of servings: varies (1 8" x 4" loaf)

Ingredients:

1 ½ cups all-purpose gluten free flour
3 medium ripe (or slightly overripe) bananas, mashed
2 large eggs
½ cup plain Greek yogurt
½ cup flax meal
½ cup unsalted butter, softened at room temperature
1 tbsp baking powder
2 tsp vanilla extract
½ tsp baking soda
½ tsp salt
¾ tsp each guar gum and xanthan gum (if your flour doesn't contain this already)
cooking spray

Preparation:

Preheat your oven to 375 F. Lightly coat a 8" x 4" loaf pan with cooking spray. Combine the dry ingredients in a large bowl with a whisk to combine. Cream the butter and sugar until fluffy in a separate bowl, then beat in the eggs until combined. Fold in the vanilla extract and yogurt. Add the dry ingredients to the butter mixture and beat until just combined. Add the mashed bananas and stir to combine. The batter should be thick and chunky.

Transfer the batter to your prepared loaf pan and smooth the top of the loaf with a spatula. Bake for 25 minutes, then tent the loaf pan with foil and continue baking for 1 hour, or until a toothpick inserted into the middle of the loaf comes out clean. Remove from the oven and allow to cool to room temperature before slicing and serving.

Buckwheat Pancakes

Number of servings: 12

Ingredients:

2 cups buckwheat flour
2 large eggs, beaten
1/3 cup powdered sugar
2 cups milk or almond milk
3 tbsp ricotta cheese
2 tbsp melted butter
1 tsp baking powder
a pinch of salt
a little oil, for cooking

Preparation:

Combine all of the ingredients in a mixing bowl and whisk together until smooth (but not totally smooth). Heat a little oil in a heavy skillet over medium heat. Once the oil is hot, add a little of the batter and cook until bubbles stop forming on the top. Flip and cook the other side until golden brown. Transfer to a plate and cover to keep warm. Repeat the process until the batter is used up. Serve hot with the toppings of your choice.

Desserts

Gluten Free Pecan Pie

Number of servings: 6 - 8

Ingredients:

The crust:
1 egg, lightly beaten
12 tbsp cold butter, cubed (1 ½ sticks of butter)
1 cup finely ground brown rice flour
½ cup arrowroot powder
½ cup amaranth flour
¼ cup white rice flour
1 tbsp brown sugar or turbinado sugar
1 tbsp very cold water
¼ tsp salt

Preparation:

Add the dry ingredients to a large mixing bowl and whisk to combine, then transfer to a food processor. Add the butter and pulse until the mixture takes on the texture of coarse crumbs. Add the egg and pulse until just incorporated. Add the water and pulse a few times to combine. If the dough doesn't hold together, add a little more water, ¼ tsp at a time until it can be formed into a ball.

Transfer the dough to a clean work surface lined with waxed paper. Flatten into a large disk. Wrap in wax paper and refrigerate for 1 – 2 hours before rolling out into a 10" circle between two sheets of waxed paper. Preheat your oven to 350 F. Carefully flip the dough into a 9" pie tin and press in to form a crust. Trim the edges and crimp with a fork. Pierce the crust in several places with a fork and bake for about 15 minutes or until golden brown. Remove from the oven and allow to cool while you make the filling.

The filling:
2 large eggs
1 cup pecans, plus extra pecan halves for topping the pie
2/3 cup sugar
½ cup light corn syrup
2 tbsp melted butter
1 tsp vanilla extract
½ tsp salt

Preparation:

Preheat your oven to 425 F. Add the eggs, corn syrup, butter, salt, vanilla extract and sugar to a food processor and pulse to combine. Add the pecans and pulse until the pecans are coarsely chopped. Pour the filling into the crust and top with pecan halves. Bake for 15 minutes, then reduce heat to 350 F and bake for another 30 minutes or until lightly browned. Remove from the oven and allow to cool on a wire rack before slicing and serving.

Gluten Free Chocolate Chip Cookies

Number of servings:

Ingredients:

3 cups almond flour
½ cup chocolate chips
½ cup butter, softened at room temperature
½ cup sugar
¼ cup chopped walnuts (this is optional, can be omitted if desired)
2 large eggs
2 tsp vanilla extract
½ tsp salt
½ tsp baking soda

Preparation:

Start by preheating your oven to 350 F. Cream the butter and sugar in a large bowl. Fold in the eggs and mix to combine. Add the baking soda, salt, almond flour and vanilla extract, then mix well. Fold in the chocolate chips and walnuts, if you're using them in this recipe. Scoop 1 tbsp of dough per cookie onto a foil lined baking sheet and bake for 12 – 14 minutes. Remove from the oven and allow to cool before serving.

Pumpkin Cake

Number of servings: varies

Ingredients:

The cake:
1 cup of canned pumpkin
3 large or extra-large eggs
1 (15 ounce) package of gluten free yellow cake mix
½ cup of canola oil
¼ cup of turbinado sugar
3 tbsp of orange juice
1 tbsp of cinnamon
2 tsp of vanilla extract
¼ tsp of ground ginger
¼ tsp of ground cloves
cooking spray
The glaze:
1 cup of powdered sugar
2 tbsp orange juice

Preparation:

Start by preheating your oven to 350 F. Lightly coat a
bundt pan with cooking spray and dust with cinnamon;
shake out the excess. Add the yellow cake mix, canned

pumpkin, sugar, orange juice, vanilla extract, eggs, ginger, remaining cinnamon and cloves to a large mixing bowl. Beat until well combined using an electric mixer or egg beater. Pour the batter into your prepared bundt pan.

Bake for 40 minutes and remove from the oven. Allow to cool for 10 – 15 minutes. Free the cake from the pan by running a thin, sharp knife around the edges of the cake. Invert the bundt pan over a wire rack and shake gently to remove the cake from the bundt pan. Allow the cake to cook completely on a wire rack (this will take at least 20 minutes). While the cake is cooling, you can make the glaze by whisking together the powdered sugar and orange juice in a small bowl. Spoon the glaze over the cake, slice and serve.

No-Bake Strawberry Pie

Number of servings: 6 – 8

Ingredients:

1 9" gluten free graham cracker pie crust
3 cups of strawberry yogurt
2 cups of sliced fresh strawberries
¾ cup of heavy cream
6 tbsp turbinado sugar
2 tsp of vanilla extract
½ tsp salt

Preparation:

Add the heavy cream, 3 tbsp of sugar and 1 tsp of vanilla extract to a mixing bowl and whisk until stiff peaks form in the mixture. Set aside. In a separate medium sized mixing bowl, add the strawberry yogurt, the other 3 tbsp of sugar, the other 1 tsp of vanilla extract and the salt. Stir until the sugar is dissolved.

Add the whipped cream and fold in to blend. Add the sliced strawberries and fold in. Transfer the mixture to the graham cracker crust and smooth the top of the pie with a spatula. Transfer the pie to the freezer and freeze until firm. Cover the pie with plastic wrap once completely frozen. When you're ready to serve the pie, remove it from the freezer and allow it to thaw for about 10 minutes before slicing and serving.

Pistachio Cheesecake

Number of servings: 6 - 8

Ingredients:

1 ¼ cups of gluten free flour
1 stick of unsalted butter
3 cups of milk
2 small packages of instant pistachio pudding
1 cup of cream cheese, softened at room temperature
1 cup of powdered sugar
1 cup of whipped topping (or make your own whipped cream)
½ cup of chopped pistachio nuts

Preparation:

The crust will take longer to make, so start by putting this together. Preheat your oven to 350 F. Melt the butter and blend with the gluten free flour and pecans in a food processor until it forms a crumbly dough like consistency. Spread the dough in a 9" x 13" baking dish and bake for 15 – 20 minutes, or until the crust becomes a light golden brown. Remove the crust from the oven and allow it to cool completely.

Now you can make the filling for your cheesecake. Mix together the softened cream cheese and the powdered sugar, then fold in half of the whipped topping or whipped cream. Spread the mixture on top of the crust once it has cooled to room temperature. Transfer to the refrigerator and chill for at least 30 minutes.

Next, mix the pistachio pudding mix with 3 cups of milk and beat for about 2 minutes or until it starts to thicken. Pour the pudding on top of the cooled crust and cream cheese filling. Return to the refrigerator and chill until the pudding has completely set. Top with the remaining whipped topping or whipped cream, slice and serve.

Brownies with Matcha

Number of servings: varies

Ingredients:

1 egg
½ cup of brown rice flour
¼ cup of white rice flour
¼ cup of tapioca flour
¼ cup butter
¼ cup (2 ounces) of unsweetened chocolate
¼ cup of dark chocolate chips
1/3 cup of turbinado sugar or sucanat
1/3 cup of coconut sugar
½ cup of coconut milk
3 tbsp of coconut milk
1 tsp baking powder
1 tsp vanilla extract
½ tsp salt
matcha powder*
cooking spray
* this is finely ground, powdered green tea. You can find matcha powder in Asian markets as well as in many larger grocery stores in the coffee and tea section.

Preparation:

Start by preheating your oven to 350 F. Melt the chocolate and butter in a double boiler over low heat. Once the chocolate and butter are melted, remove from heat and allow it to cool slightly. Lightly coat a 8" x 8" square pan with cooking spray and set aside.

Combine all of the dry ingredients in a large mixing bowl. Add the egg, vanilla extract and milk. Beat with an electric hand mixer or egg beater. When combined, add the chocolate and butter mixture. Beat at high speed until the batter is well mixed and creamy in texture.

Pour the batter into your prepared cake pan. Sprinkle the chocolate chips over the top of the brownies evenly and allow them to sink into the batter. Place the brownies in the oven and bake for 30 minutes, or until a toothpick inserted into the center comes out clean. Remove the brownies from the oven and allow them to cool in the pan. While the brownies are cooling, dust the top with matcha powder and cool to room temperature before slicing and serving.

Gluten Free Weight Loss Conclusion

The recipes in this book are meant to provide you with a good introduction to the gluten free lifestyle, whether your plan is to eliminate it from your diet for a shorter term weight loss or maintenance plan or to make a lifelong habit of eating a diet which does not contain this often problematic protein. By cooking these meals, you'll begin to get a feeling for how you can create meals without gluten and along the way, come up with some new gluten free recipes of your own.

As with any cookbook, you should feel free to experiment a little with the recipes. If you think a dish would benefit from a different herb, more or less garlic or so on, go right ahead – you're the chef here, after all. If you're less experienced in the kitchen, then you may want to follow these recipes as they are written until you gain a little confidence in your culinary skills, however.

Other than weight loss and better health, one of the biggest benefits of going on a diet like the gluten free diet is that it allows you to get a new perspective on cooking and can help you to become a more skilled and creative cook, which is never a bad thing. From appetizers to desserts, breakfast to dinner, there is almost nothing that you can't make gluten free; and of course, there are probably many foods which you already enjoy that contain no gluten – include these in your diet as well, provided that they follow the basic guideline of being as unprocessed as possible and of course, nutritious. Once you get gluten out of your life and learn how to live (and cook) without it, you may never go back again, even if you don't have a sensitivity to this common protein.

CPSIA information can be obtained
at www.ICGtesting.com
Printed in the USA
BVHW040204140422
634326BV00016B/281